BODY
BLUEPRINT

How Your Pain May be Telling a Story

JODI SCHOLES

JODI SCHOLES
Speaker · Educator · Bodyworker

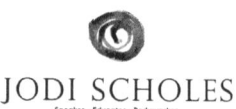

JODI SCHOLES
Speaker · Educator · Bodyworker

DEDICATION

I dedicate this book to the people experiencing pain.
To the people who suffer from a mysterious illness,
whose doctor tells them the tests were negative and
there is no clinical reason for their symptoms.
There is a reason.
To healthy folks, too, who are curious about
how their body works.
For each of you.

with love,

Jodi

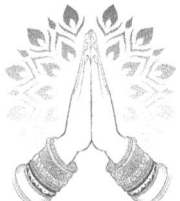

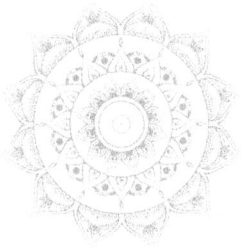

FOREWORD

Who do you know who lives in daily pain? If it's not you, then it's someone you know because you picked up this book. The Centers for Disease Control (CDC) reports that pain compromises the lives of over 50 million people in the United States. And over 20 million of those people have high-impact pain, meaning pain that interferes daily with their lives.[1] In 2016, pain cost the United States about $635,000,000,000. That number reads, with *b*, 635 billion dollars.

I wrote this book for you, the person who questions the reasons for pain. The seeker of knowledge. The person ready to investigate to find the cause of the pain, even if the breadcrumbs lead back to themselves. This book is for the person willing to look at the dis-ease in their lives. It is for the adventurer who wants to explore the mountains and valleys of their soul.

The following quote may look familiar. It's a classic. Psalm 23 talks about the dark days:

> *The Lord is my shepherd, I lack nothing.*
> *He makes me lie down in green pastures,*
> *He leads me beside quiet waters. He refreshes my soul.*

He guides me along the right paths for his name's sake.
Even though I walk through the darkest valley,
I will fear no evil, for you are with me;
your rod and your staff, they comfort me.
You prepare a table before me in the presence of my enemies.
You anoint my head with oil; my cup overflows.
Surely your goodness and love will follow me all the days of my life,
and I will dwell in the house of the LORD forever. (NIV)

You may encounter a few dark valleys in the pages of this book. We will visit, or perhaps revisit, some experiences and difficulties you may have ignored or never even considered. Sometimes, it may be uncomfortable, but I promise this trek is worth every step. We are exploring beyond the obvious to identify what may be causing your pain. If you feel some resistance, that's normal. The answers you deserve are just below the surface, and over the following pages of this book, we will go there together.

Since we will walk this path together, I invite you to share your stories. I'm on most of the social media channels, but if IG messages or FB DMs aren't your thing, I encourage you to email me from my website www.jodischoles.com. I *love* reading your insights and successes in identifying and releasing pain!

Today, we begin the journey of discovering *your* unique story. It's serious work, but the stories told here may let us laugh a little along the way. Even if it's just a chuckle, acknowledging we are not alone. Stage actress Ethel Barrymore said, "You grow up the day you have the first good laugh at yourself." We may be on a bumpy ride, but let's agree not to take ourselves too seriously.

This journey is life-changing work because, by eliminating all the sources of your pain, we make room for more joy. What I believe and see for you is a pain-free, healthy, vibrant version of yourself.

By the end of this book, you will discover some surprising answers as to what causes pain and what to do about it. I'm betting that you have a sense in your gut that there is a solution for what you are experiencing right now. You sense there is an ah-ha moment just over the horizon. Like the miners of old sensing that there is gold in them thar hills, you know you are getting close to your answers.

Stubborn pain has a story to tell. We can't just treat the symptoms. Well, we can, but too often, when we do, the pain remains. Thank you for picking up this book. I am honored to be here with you. You are in the right place.

Let's do this.

Jodi Scholes

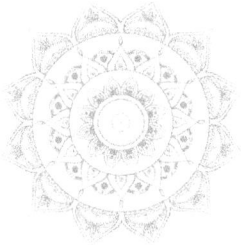

ACKNOWLEDGMENTS

To my friends and family in Northern Virginia, Florida, and New Hampshire - thank you for your patience, encouragement, and support while writing this book. Here it is. Finally.

There's no way I would have lasted with pro soccer, through four MLS championships, a few thousand hours of locker room treatments, and countless road trips, without the camaraderie and appreciation of the medical team and training staff at D.C. United, a Washington D.C. based professional soccer team. While working for ten years as a Licensed Massage Therapist with this team, I had the great fortune to work with top-notch medical professional colleagues. I tip my hat to Rick Guter, Head Athletic Trainer and Physical Therapist, who officially invited me to join the team. Thank you to Rick's contemporary, Brian "Goody' Goodstein, ATC, for keeping me on the team. Thank you to orthopedic surgeons Dr. Bill Hazel, MD, and Dr. Chris Annunziata, MD, Dr. Emilio Canal, DDS who shared their decades of experience with me as well as appreciated how massage therapy positively impacted the rehab and recovery of professional athletes. I am grateful to Dr. Hirad Bagey, D.C., for teaching me about the importance of working with the ankles and feet. I deeply respect my colleague Jenni Roberts, LMT, for being my enthusiastic partner in the locker room. We were the only two females amidst this band of brothers.

Thank you to Bonnie Vining and the rest of the Vining family, who have generously allowed me to include my client, Jim Vining's World War II experience in his own words, which he typed on his electric typewriter.

Thank you to Kristen White, for the coaching and support to land my TEDx talk. In her intuitive wisdom, she insisted I write a book.

Thank you to Keren Kilgore for her tireless patience in getting this book over the finish line.

And finally, thank you to my friend Michelle Bendel Donahue for listening to me drone on about this book and the marathon edit we did together. You, the reader, can be grateful to MBD, too. This book is way better after being reviewed by her keen eyes and compassionate clarity.

Disclosure

This book is not a substitute for traditional Western medicine. It is meant to work hand in hand with the orthodox medicine you've known all your life. If you are experiencing sharp shooting pain in your gut because you think your appendix is about to burst, the message is clear: Go to the Emergency Room.

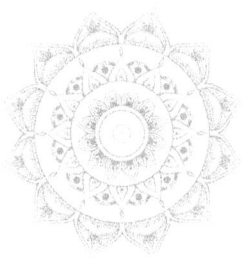

CONTENTS

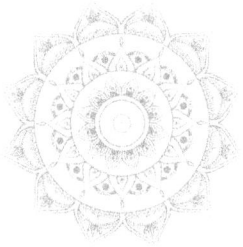

INTRODUCTION

These pains you feel are messengers. Listen to them.

~ Rumi

Biography Becomes Biology

Over the next few pages, we will consider how your biography, the story of your life, affects your biology—your health and well-being. We will investigate how *what you believe, what you tell yourself, and what you experience as the truth* affects your physical body. We generally know stress can have adverse effects on your health. But what if you knew exactly how specific stressors affected you?

Consider this book your cheat sheet. It will guide you to discover where specific types of stress appear in your body and how they manifest. Let's look at some examples.

Broken Heart Syndrome

Scientists are now studying Takotsubo syndrome, also known as Broken Heart Syndrome or Cardiomyopathy. Johnny Cash died four months after his beloved wife of 35 years, June Carter Cash. Friends close to the legendary singer say Johnny died of a broken heart.

Did you know that Debbie Reynolds, the Singin' in the Rain star, loved Christmas so much that she kept a tree up all year? Her daughter, Carrie Fisher, Princess Leia in Star Wars, knew this and planned to travel from London to Los Angeles to spend the holidays with her mom. You might have seen the tabloid stories about their turbulent relationship, filled with intense fights but also unwavering loyalty over the years.

In December 2016, Debbie planned the menu and set the dinner table with the Christmas pattern China plates. On December 23, Carrie was making the 11-hour flight when she suffered a massive heart attack. She was treated and spent Christmas Day in the hospital. She died a few days later, on December 27, 2016. What is unusual about this story is that Debbie Reynolds, her grief-stricken mom, died just one day later, on 28 Dec 2016. During the hours that followed Carrie's death, Debbie's son remembers his mother repeating out loud that she just wanted to be with her daughter.

Former British Prime Minister (1976-1979), James Callaghan was married to his sweetheart, Audrey, for 66 years. Eleven days after Audrey passed away, having no previous health conditions, he died suddenly.

Is it an urban legend that couples married for many years often die within days, weeks, or months of each other? A study from the National Library of Medicine called Patterns of Widowhood says, "Death of a spouse is associated with an increased age-specific probability of dying for the surviving spouse.... Widowhood disrupts long-standing companionship and social support patterns and entails financial adjustments and other major lifestyle modifications. Adapting to these changes may lead to poor health outcomes for the surviving spouse."[2]

Muscle Memory

"Do you want a tissue?" I asked. About 20 minutes into her session, my client Betsy started to cry.

It wasn't a normal reaction to my massage. I was curious about what she was experiencing. Was it a physical response, or had I inadvertently caused emotional upheaval? A memory had popped into her head. She said it felt like she was there again, sitting on the floor in her kitchen with her back against the cupboards, her knees tucked under her chin, and her husband kicking her.

She couldn't remember what she had done wrong. It wasn't the first time her husband had physically beaten her, but it was one of the last times. She told me she divorced this man and is doing some much-needed self-care. She admitted she spent too many years in an abusive relationship. During the session, the nurturing touch to her lower leg allowed this old, buried memory to surface. This experience is an example of muscle memory. After a long exhale, she told me she was fine continuing the session. With her permission, we forged ahead.

Her body had healed from those bruises years before, but her emotions at the time of the abuse had been denied, ignored, and buried. As a result, her emotional body was still wounded. She remembered telling herself things like *Just move on. He didn't mean it. He won't do it again. He said he was sorry. It wasn't that bad.*

But it was that bad. And she finally had the courage to leave. She was brave and made a difficult change. I believe the tears were shed for her past self and what she endured.

This autonomic body response could also be called a Somatic Emotional Release. I didn't intend to release any trauma from her body. I'm pretty sure my client didn't intend to cry. However, this client was healing on many levels - physically, mentally, and emotionally. Sometimes, our physical body has healed, but our emotions still need time to recover.

Pain sends us a message that something needs to heal physically, mentally, or emotionally. Muscle memory is another example of how our biography affects our biology.

The Big Stick

I wanted one last run down the mountain. Just as I reached the bottom of the last hill, the snowboard shot out from under me. I hit the ground so hard that my teeth clunked together. I stared at the late afternoon sky lying on the frozen ground. Slowly, I rolled over. I carefully got to my knees. How did I fall so hard so fast? Eventually, I stood, brushed off the snow, lifted my arms, and ran my tongue across my teeth. Check. My brisk body scan determined nothing was broken. But I had a feeling I'd be sore from that little episode.

The two-hour drive home stretched into three hours as I watched the bright red taillights in stop-and-go traffic. Hey, a tough day on the mountain was still more fun than a long day at the office. I'd been out of massage school for less than a year. I was the owner of a brand-new, barely furnished massage clinic with no time for days off. I'd have the entire night to recover.

The following day, my coworker saw me gingerly walking down the hallway. I saw her eyebrows lift in a question mark.

"I'm good," I assured her with a thumbs up. "As long as I move slowly."

She remained unconvinced as I tried to hobble down the hallway. "Look," she called after me, "you're feeling this pain for a reason."

That hadn't occurred to me. I knew why I was in pain but had not considered that the pain was trying to get my attention.

"If you ignore it…" she started.

"Fat chance of that," I laughed. My back felt like a big stick had whacked it.

"If you ignore pain," she said, interrupting me, "it will tap you on the shoulder, and if that doesn't work, then it will knock you up the side of your head."

As she walked away, I heard her ask, "What if this is the tap? What is it trying to teach you?"

What if *this* pain was the tap? Yikes. Was pain tap, tap, tapping to get my attention? I paused to think. When I asked myself what's the message in this pain, I realized I rarely gave myself permission to listen to my body. I always pushed through. I always played the role of a superhero. The serious pain I was experiencing was trying to give me permission to rest. The pain told me I was vulnerable, and the lesson was that it's okay to chill now and then.

Total Pain

Consider the pioneering English physician Dame Cicely Saunders. She created what we know today as Hospice Care in the 1950s. Hospice is a specific type of palliative care at the end of life. Dame Cicely's research on managing symptoms at the end of life led her to introduce the world to the term "Total Pain."

"Total Pain" is the many facets of pain her patients experience at the end of their lives, not just physical but social, spiritual, and psychological/emotional. Her research showed some Hospice patients get depressed. Some feel regret or remorse. Some wonder about what is to come next. Some worry and are deeply saddened to be leaving their family behind. Dame Cicely looked beyond pharmacological solutions. At St. Christopher's Hospital, the research results, measured on the same 1 to 10 pain scale still in use, showed that when someone was present to listen, care, and sit with the patient, even in silence, many patients reported they felt less pain. The point is to ease patients' pain with medicine as their physical condition worsens. But at the end of life, we must consider the concept of Total Pain, which can involve the patient's mental and emotional state.

Pain Is an Honest Friend

Here's the big secret of my book: *There's a message in the pain.* It's like you receive a telegram from the universe in the form of pain. Imagine your phone ringing.

You answer, "Hello?"

"Hi, this is the universe calling. I have a message for you."

Suddenly, you feel a stabbing pain in the lower back. The message is coming in the form of pain. Most people say, "Wrong number," and hang up the phone. How about you? Do you disconnect, ignore the pain, and soldier on?

Or are you curious?

After working with 20,000 clients, my experience and research show there is almost always a message in the pain. In the pages of this book, you can read the present-day messages pain is sending. But pain has been sending tap-tap telegrams for thousands of years.

Pain taps you on the shoulder, saying, "Slow down. No need to work so hard."

Perhaps pain taps your knee. "End that toxic relationship."

Pain taps your neck with a sore throat, whispering, "Find and use your voice."

Pain is telling a story. Pain is telling *your* story. It is telling the story we don't dare to tell ourselves. Pain is telling us it's time to change something in our life. Pain is not the enemy. It is like an honest friend. Pain is not here to sabotage our lives but to interrupt our lives, to get our attention. Then we have to pay attention.

So, how do we figure out the message?

Once we understand the location and origin of the pain, we can consider its purpose. We will use ancient wisdom combined with my decades of experience and hands-on research to interpret *your Body Blueprint* in the present day. In doing so, we will explore the origins of pain and the many layers of internal and external causes that show up as physical pain.

Doctors Don't Have All the Answers

Recently, a professional race car driver asked me, "Why doesn't my doctor talk about this?"

That's a loaded question. Though there are many wonderful triumphs, there are also many challenges with the healthcare system in the United States. Western medicine is almost always singularly focused on the physical causes of pain. We are about to learn that the causes of pain are not just physical. So, how do we figure it out?

Spoiler alert: There is no magic formula. No cookie-cutter solution.

Your story is unique and all your own, so you get to explore *your* truth based on your biography. The good news is there is a road map, an ancient Body Blueprint, that gives us clues. And when we pay attention, we can uncover the answers. The Body

Blueprint helps us heal physical pain by considering the mental suffering and emotional aches that want our attention.

It's easy to recognize when we are in physical pain. To understand chronic pain (pain that comes back repeatedly), we must explore our history. Perhaps most of the time, your pain is situational, meaning you know the cause. (Like a tough workout with a personal trainer, packing up and moving boxes all day, or a long hike on hilly terrain.) *Chronic pain,* however, often originates in three areas at once: physical, mental, and emotional. This is the founding principle of the Biopsychosocial Model.

The what?

The Bio.Psycho.Social model.

The Biopsychosocial Model

In 1977, Dr. George Engel introduced the Biopsychosocial Model to several of his medical colleagues at the University of Rochester in New York. He was a professor of both Psychology and Medicine. He published on hundreds of occasions, writings about the connection between emotions and disease. Practically speaking, his concern was that medicine was becoming too focused on technology and too distant from the patient. He believed the doctor's bedside manner had turned cold and impersonal. He encouraged doctors to examine the patient honestly. To consider their biological condition, the patient's psychology (mental stress), and social pressures affecting the patient. He taught doctors to ask about external circumstances contributing to the patient's experience of pain in addition to ordering blood tests and MRIs. He wanted medical professionals to remember the importance of connecting with patients by talking to them.

How logical, right?

The National Institutes of Health defines the Biopsychosocial Model as "Philosophically, it is a way of understanding how suffering, disease, and illness are affected by multiple levels of the organization, from the societal to the molecular." [3] The British Medical Journal says, "In spite of the traditional dominance of the biomedical model, the time seems right for expanding the model to the Biopsychosocial Model as the social and psychological influences of today's health problems do not fit the narrow framework of the biomedical model."[4]

One more shout-out for Dr. Engel. He said, "We are now faced with the necessity and the challenge to broaden the approach to disease to include the psychosocial without sacrificing the enormous advantages of the biomedical approach."[5] Dr. Engel's "now" was 1979.

CHAPTER 1

THE JAW

Our lives begin to end the day we become silent
about things that matter.

~ Martin Luther King Jr.

What Goes Unsaid - Grace

Grace rubbed the sides of her face slowly, closing her eyes. She looked pale and tired. Travel during the holidays had taken a lot out of her. She was grateful she had planned a massage between Christmas and the New Year.

By the time she arrived for her massage, Grace admitted she had been sipping her meals through a straw for two days. Well, that's not normal. I asked if this had happened before. She was glib but somber, "Eh, it happens now and then." Trying to deflect the ridiculousness of the situation, she joked about good news and bad news. Good news: the last time this happened, she tried

Kate Farms Vanilla Nutrition Shake instead of the old standby Ensure. Kate Farms was delicious; bonus, she still had some in the pantry. The bad news was her husband grilled burgers and corn on the cob the night before. It smelled delicious, but she couldn't open her mouth wide enough to take a bite.

Grace's family visit had been stressful. In the past, family gatherings were always full of gossip about relatives. Cousin Louie was getting a divorce. Uncle Dan hasn't spoken to his son in over six months. Grace would stay quiet as the stories swirled. She observed. She didn't like talking about people. She preferred to talk about past vacations, current hobbies, boho jewelry, or a favorite book. So many other topics. She didn't like gossip, but she didn't like confrontation either. Her mantra was, "Silence is golden." It is, until it's not.

The pressure had started before the trip. It was an election year, and the calls with her family had been tense. Grace is middle of the road in her political views. Her older sister, a fiery Leo, is decidedly more liberal.

Grace guessed the jaw pain had started around the time her sister provoked her mom saying something to the effect, "That's what you get. You voted for him."

She said her stomach flipped when her mom shot back a retort about how she has a right to an opinion, and her vote counts just as much as anyone else. She said she'd be willing to stand in line for hours to vote if it would cancel out her eldest daughter's bad decisions.

Grace bit her lip and stayed silent. She didn't like the way her sister provoked her mother. Nor her mother's characteristic offensive defense. But Grace doesn't like confrontation.

Sandpaper People

Family can be tough. There are some people who I believe are put on this Earth to be sandpaper. Sandpaper? Yes, I call them

Sandpaper People. What do we know about sandpaper? The abrasive material changes the surface of anything it encounters. Sandpaper makes things smoother, but it does so by wearing down an external layer. That's the job of the Sandpaper People in our lives. They wear down our patience and expose the vulnerabilities and rawness underneath.

We can learn to be grateful for Sandpaper People. Yes, the people who annoy us the most are the best teachers in our lives. When abrasive comments rub us the wrong way, it can be a sign to look inside ourselves. It's not about them; it's always about us. We take our power back by asking, "Ok, what am I making this mean?" How do you recognize Sandpaper People? They create psychological stress and socially tense situations. When they enter a room, you will notice a physical shift in your body. Maybe your lips purse or you fold your arms around yourself. Grace clenched her jaw, which locked down her urge to speak.

This is an all-too-common reaction for women. Brene Brown writes, "Even to me the issue of 'stay small, sweet, quiet, and modest' sounds like an outdated problem, but the truth is that women still run into those demands whenever we find and use our voices."[6]

Jaw pain is often about holding back communication. To help relieve jaw pain, how can one find and use the voice? I've had clients who decided to scream into a pillow, one took singing lessons and joined the church choir. It sounds crazy, but speaking out loud is like training a muscle. When you have regular time to express yourself out loud, you start to express yourself out loud more easily and more often.

Geek alert: Stress and TMJ

A recent study by the National Journal of Maxillofacial Surgery found, "Stress is a significant etiologic factor involved in initiation and maintenance of TMJDs in dental students."[7] This quote means we clench our jaws in times of stress. Additionally, researchers from *The Journal of Pain* evaluated 4,000 people and found those with depression and anxiety had an increased risk for Temporomandibular pain upon palpation.[8]

Dental research has also proven anger and stress correlate directly with Temporomandibular Joint Disorder (TMJD). Most likely a result of clenching the jaw. Each person has their way of processing stress. Do you grind your teeth at night? A mouth guard is one of the solutions, but not the only answer – although your dentist will be very pleased you are wearing it! Explore beyond the physical symptoms down into the layers of the issue. Ask yourself, "What is the source of the tension causing me to grind my teeth? Why am I grinding my teeth?" Then, acknowledge what rises to the top.

In her book *Heal Your Body A-Z,* Louise Hay writes the probable cause of TMJ pain is anger, resentment, and a desire for revenge. She suggests using the phrase, "I am willing to change the patterns in me that created this condition. I love and approve of myself. I am safe."[9] This is called an affirmation. Albeit helpful, we may need to take more action. Another bodyworker and author, Emily A. Francis, in her book, *The Body Heals Itself,* writes, "The jaws are the space for old pains, anguish, shame, and anger."[10] She goes on to explain words that need to be said but are never spoken can get stored in the jaw.

By the way, clenching teeth can be felt and seen. The tension is revealed in body language without ever saying a word. Did you know humans can detect the muscles of the jaw clenching even if the muscles of the face don't move? Research says we can *feel it* intuitively. Your spouse/partner can feel it. So can your kid. So, you're busted. Even though the clench may help you avoid using words as weapons, it can also hurt you by causing Temporomandibular joint (TMJ) jaw pain.

The Lesson: Say What Needs to Be Said

The first step to getting rid of jaw pain is to acknowledge the conversations you have muted. Say what needs to be said. You don't have to say it directly to the person. You can role-play the conversation. It can be advantageous if the person is not present - at least they won't interrupt you! Saying words out loud will start the process of relieving the psychological component of jaw pain.

If that doesn't relieve the clenching or if it comes back, we can explore the emotion of anger. What are you angry about? What would you say to that person? If you want to skip the conversation, go directly to step two: Forgiveness.

This jaw pain is getting your attention for a reason. You are learning that harboring anger can cause pain or make you sick. Yes, it's making your jaw hurt, but dis-ease in the body can turn into disease.

⌐ The Exercise: Three Parts ⌐

Part One

In what current situation do you feel you have lost your voice? What words would you say now? Consider saying these phrases before bed or when you feel less than powerful:

I am worthy.

What I say is important.

I trust myself.

I am safe.

My voice matters.

I love, and I am loveable.

I speak my truth.

All is well.

To keep it simple, start with one positive phrase. Pick from the ones listed here or make your own. Other practices that can help with the stress of feeling disempowered include:

Meditation - Apps, classes, quiet time

Breathing exercises - Transformational breathwork

Walking in nature

Positive visualization

Part Two

Think about your jaw pain. Is it the left side, right side, or bilateral (both)? If your pain is one-sided, it represents either male or female energy. The right represents the masculine. Make a note of that. We have already mentioned that jaw pain is about communication.

Right side pain? Ask, *Is there a man (masculine energy) I need to talk to?*

Left side pain? Ask, *Is there a female (feminine energy) I need to talk to?*

Bilateral pain? Ask, *What family member, neighbor, or coworker do I need to talk to?*

Jaw pain can also be about anger, resentment, and revenge.

Make some more notes:

Who do you resent?

Who are you angry with? (maybe with yourself, but who else?)

Who do you feel deserves revenge?

Consider how your jaw feels when you chew.

What am I chewing on over and over?

What am I not willing to assimilate?

What am I not willing to take in?

If no answers to any of these questions readily come to mind, that's okay. As you go to bed, ask your subconscious mind to think about it; then ask yourself again when you wake up in the morning. It's helpful to ask yourself questions within the first hour of waking up. In the morning, your mind is fresh and not polluted with the distractions of the day. You are less likely to resist. Make it a game. Play with the answers. There is a very good possibility you do know where this pain is coming from. You're just not aware of it yet.

For you A+ overachievers, feeling stuck and not getting clear answers can cause some frustration, I have one last suggestion: Ask a friend.

Explain that you are doing some self-reflection, and you want their opinion. "Who do you think I am angry with?" "Who do I resent?" "Who would I love to get revenge on?" Friends remember everything. Long after you've buried the anger, they'll tell you what they remember.

Part Three

Think of a time in your life when you *didn't* say what you wanted to say. Pause. Breathe. Think. Something coming to mind?

1. Grab a timer, a pen, and some paper. Find a quiet spot away from others. Even the bathroom will do.

2. In your chosen quiet place, shut the door and sit down.

3. Set the timer for seven minutes.

4. Breathe. Listen to your breath. Count 1-2-3 on the inhale. Count 1-2-3 on the exhale. Slow it down.

5. Ask yourself, *When was a time in my life when I wanted to say something and didn't?* Sit there. What or who comes to mind? Jot down any words that pop into your head. Any person. Consider that there may be more than one.

6. Ask yourself, *What else do you want me to know about my jaw pain?* Consider that there may be additional guidance from your angels, the universe, intuition, or the God of your understanding.

7. What words did you jot down? Did you get an answer you understand? If not, no big deal. We are going to investigate a bit more. This next step might be your favorite part.

8. The next step in getting rid of this jaw pain is to have a conversation with the person you need to speak with. It can be in person or *in your imagination* but speak your words out loud. Even if it seems off the wall, the words spoken will inform your subconscious of the event. Imagination is a powerful tool. Let's use it to release the pain using words. How does that work? Set a time and a place. For example, on Friday night, pour yourself a tall glass of your favorite adult beverage or make a nice cup of tea and have a chat. Role play. Have a talk. It's what your body needs to release some of the jaw tension. The idea is to act as if they are sitting in the chair next to you and then you can express your feelings to them.

At some weddings, a chair is left empty in the front row for the spirit of a departed loved one to sit. Likewise, if you are invited to a bris, an empty chair is set for the prophet Elijah. He is said to oversee every ceremony when summoned, bringing protection and peace.

Even if the person you want to talk with isn't in the room, you can still have the conversation. If you have ever prayed, then you may be comfortable talking to someone who isn't physically in front of you. If you're not the praying type, I'd encourage you to experiment. Some say praying is talking to God, and meditation is listening to God. The answers that arrive may look a little different than you could have imagined.

Additional Note

My parents used to tell me G.I.G.O. Garbage In, Garbage Out. Through my interactions with numerous clients, I have come across a prevailing issue: stress induced by constant exposure to news reporting stimuli. The never-ending 24-7 news cycle tends to generate persistent low-grade stress for virtually anyone within the sound of its buzz and bewilderment. Like the din of the ear ringing with tinnitus, if the TV is on, constant background noise reminds us of what's going wrong. Gun violence in shopping malls and schools, political mudslinging: She's awful; He's a liar; military clashes on the border; natural disasters like earthquakes and hurricanes. There is rarely *good news* being reported. Consider testing this theory by taking a 24-hour break from the news.

Oh my! Turn off the TV and notifications. (gasp) Yes. It will be there if/when you come back. Take a 24-hour break and see if your jaw pain changes. Stop watching TV before and while you go to sleep. No TV playing in the bedroom during sleeping time? Why? The tone of the commentary on the TV registers in your brain and can keep you from deep sleep. See how it feels to sleep in a quiet room. See if you get better sleep that night. If/when your jaw pain decreases, maybe that's a new option. Consider it intermittent fasting one or two days a week from the news.

The Final Step

The final step in this process is forgiveness. Forgive them? Yes. Forgive them for being stuck. Forgive them for being scared. Forgive them for saying hurtful words. Forgive them for not showing up the way you thought they should. Forgive them for not giving you the love and respect you deserve. You may not be ready, and that's okay. Maybe later. For now, forgive yourself for not being ready.

Whether the stress is physical, mental, or emotional, I take this opportunity to gently remind you, you can treat the symptoms, but that doesn't solve the problem. If you don't address the underlying cause of the stress, the condition will persist.

How would you feel about saying a prayer for the Sandpaper People in your life? No, silly goose, you don't pray for them to fail. You speak a blessing to them. Try something like, "I wish for [Sandpaper Person's name] happiness. I see [name] as healthy and perfect just the way they are. I send [name] a blessing of joy and abundance."

C H A P T E R   2

THE NECK

Every cell in your body is eavesdropping
on your thoughts.

~ Deepak Chopra

Who is Your Pain in the Neck? - Karen

As Karen stepped outside, the cold morning air made the inside of her nose freeze. Ah, winter in Maine. The snow crunched as she walked. The car door made a creaking noise that almost sounded like it was complaining it had to move. Karen wanted to let the engine warm, but the seat cushion was cold. She clicked the button to turn on the seat warmer and gently changed gears from park to reverse. All she could see were shapes through the frozen water in the rear-view camera.

That's when it happened. She turned to look behind her to back out of the driveway; she felt a sharp zing from her ear to shoulder on the right side of her neck. It was almost like an electric shock, and then came a warm feeling. She paused and put the car back into park. Pulling her hand from the glove, she slowly rubbed the right side of her neck. She thought, "Well, that came from out of nowhere."

Or did it?

Sound familiar? It does to me. I have felt that zing. Usually, when I'm rushing. When pain jolts down my neck, I slow down, take a minute, and breathe.

Sometimes, the message in the pain is that simple: slow down. Notice if you are in a hurry for no important reason. Come to the present moment.

Karen was out on this particular morning to deliver pain medicine to her 35-year-old son, who struggled with addiction. She crawled out of her warm bed to deliver the Percocet. She was not happy about it but rationalized, at *least it's not 2 am calls, where he's moaning in pain.*

Karen noticed that her neck pain disappeared when her son went to rehab (and was not her responsibility). She was unsure if it came back because of her interrupted sleep or the stress of the constant worry that he could hurt himself or someone else. It was probably a combination of both, but that's a battle she'd put off to fight another day. For now, she was off to drop off his meds.

Karen has always stepped up to take care of her family. Are you the mom or dad, bonus mom or stepdad, the responsible one in the family who solves all the problems? Are you the go-to person because you always just get it done? If so, consider for a moment what it would feel like to release that burden of responsibility. Do you daydream about disappearing? Karen did. In fact, she and her husband were planning an extended vacation on a river cruise through Europe. She read she might not have phone service on the boat and loved the idea.

Her son needed help, but was also crossing some of Karen's boundaries. Calling at all hours of the day and night. Expecting his needs to be the priority. To Karen and others, these expectations felt poor form on his part. Maybe even taking advantage of her. But at the end of the day, it was up to Karen to recognize and respect her boundaries.

The opportunity to set clear boundaries with her son presented itself sooner than anticipated. She knocked on the door. When the door opened, she could smell he'd been drinking. Without saying a word, she walked into the kitchen, put the pill on the counter, turned around, and left. Later that morning, she and her husband had *the talk*. It was time for the son to return to rehab. He agreed, suggesting, "How about after we return from the cruise?"

Karen was brave and said, "No, before we leave."

The pain in your neck could be a person who is, literally, manifesting as a pain in the neck.

Another Pain In the Neck - Ann

On a hot and muggy day in Louisiana, Ann found herself faced with a pile of work, prompting her to head to her office on a Saturday. When she arrived, she saw another car in the parking lot. The new COO (already nicknamed the Chief Obedience Officer) was also at work. Ann isn't a big fan of this guy. A short and overconfident fellow, he looked her up and down at their first meeting, making her very uncomfortable. She would avoid him if possible.

Walking into her office, she found it unbearably hot. As a woman going through menopause, she preferred it a little on the cooler side. Instantly feeling little beads of sweat on her hairline, she saw it was 78 degrees. She smiled at her body's reaction to the heat as she pressed the down arrow on the thermostat. Nothing changed. She tapped the down arrow 2 or 3 times. Nothing happened. She pressed and held the down button. Nothing. She looked over at her desk, and a paperback book's cover and back pages had started to curl. Hmmm, weird. She thought, *It's really sticky in here; I wonder if the AC is working.*

Reluctantly, she walked down to the COO's office. He barely turned his head to acknowledge she walked in. After she asked about the temperature in her office, he explained that the AC was working perfectly. He controlled the building temperature from an app on his phone and locked all the thermostats. "I've been cutting costs. Running the AC at a little higher temp when no one is in the building." Picking up his phone and punching buttons, he made it clear that he'd unlock it, but just for the day. Then, tapping the thermostat in his office, he reminded Ann to reset the temperature back to 78 degrees when she left, or he'd lock the thermostat again.

As Ann walked back to her office, unsuspectingly, anger and defensive feelings bubbled up in her torso. Am I 10 years old? His words replayed in her mind, 'Remember to adjust the thermostat or else?' What kind of communication style is that?

Seated at her desk, she propped the door open a little for airflow and waited for the space to cool off. Ann took a deep breath. She tilted her head to the side and dropped her ear to her shoulder. She heard a pop as her neck adjusted. She could feel tension running from the bottom of her skull towards her right shoulder. Each time she had an encounter with this fellow, she found she needed to pause and breathe.

Ann took a moment to ask herself, *What is it about this situation that is so irritating? Is it his attitude? His demeanor? His condescending comments?* She giggled as she considered the idea that he was overcompensating because he was nervous. It's true. All eyes are on him because he's the new guy. He's trying to make a good impression. She smiled, thinking, *A swing and a miss on that one, buddy.* Her body relaxes just a little. She sees the situation differently now. The behavior and words are still offensive. But, at least for now, she had found her way to having compassion by seeing two sides to the story.

A Brief Introduction to Masculine and Feminine Energy

To decode a more specific message associated with your neck pain, we explore our masculine and feminine nature. In her book *WomanCode*, hormone expert Alissa Vitti explains, "Both energies exist within each of us in varying amounts. Learning how to engage fully is what ends up making a person psychologically, emotionally, and physically well. Just as you wouldn't operate a remote control with only one battery, you need both of these energies as your power sources."[11]

How does the masculine and feminine nature have anything to do with neck pain? Right-side neck pain? The right side of the body represents masculine energy. Is there a male in your life you consider a pain in the neck?

Left side neck pain? The left side of the body represents feminine energy. Is there a female in your life that you consider a pain in the neck?

A brief word about bilateral neck pain. It is unusual but represents its message. Bilateral neck pain can indicate our inability to see both sides of a story. Turn your head left and then right. On what issue are you unwilling to listen to both sides of the story? Many people don't recognize when they are being stubborn. We can benefit from acknowledging there is more than one way to see a thing. When we recognize someone else's point of view, we see (not necessarily agree) both sides of the story.

In this image called Rubin's vase, what do you see? A vase? Or do you see two profiles looking at each other? Who is right? Both. This demonstrates there are sometimes two sides to a story. And neither answer is wrong.

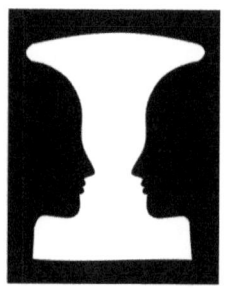

The Lesson - Identify *Your* Pain in the Neck

To understand neck pain, let's look beyond the physical reasons. Persistent neck pain allows us to ask, *Who is the pain in the neck? Who would you call a pain in the neck in your life? Is there a person in your family or work environment with whom you don't see eye to eye?*

There is a good chance the ladies in my stories have pain in their necks because of a person acting like a pain in the neck. Is it a coincidence that neck pain worsens when dealing with a specific person? No, it isn't. But what can be done? Control what you can control in your own life. Chaos in someone else's life doesn't translate to mean chaos in your life.

Have you heard the term, *not my monkey, not my circus*? Make space (and sometimes distance) from those who create chaos in their lives. Hopefully, you don't have chaos in your home or at work. But if you have chronic neck pain, your pain in the neck likely has a first and last name programmed into your phone.

Depending on what state of mind you are in, we could take the high road here. Could you find compassion for them? In the story, Angela found her way to have compassion. Of course, you often have the opportunity to pause to look in the mirror and identify your part of the conflict. Owning your part doesn't justify their bad behavior. The time to pause will often give you a new point of reference. A point of view that could provide some patience and help to relieve the neck pain.

Just like our pain can illuminate the story, *our words* often dictate the story. Let's look at language. These are such common statements:

Jeez, he's breathing down my neck!
I broke my neck to get all the work done on time.
The Director of Operations is such a pain in the neck.

Be careful with the words you choose. You may be manifesting your own pain. These declarations slip out of the mouth without a second thought. Choose words carefully. We create what we declare. Quite literally, words have a vibration. Vibration is energy. When we speak words intentionally, out loud, that is the start of creating a reality. If you want to get relief from the pain in your neck, *stop using words* that create that reality.

Rephrasing ideas.

Jeez, he's asked three times for that report!
I spent hours over the weekend working on the project to get all the work done on time.
The Director of Operations micromanages every project in the office.

Here's another simple example of words being a creative force from ordinary life. When a parent warns a child, saying, "Oh, be careful, you are going to spill that!" That parent has just painted the picture of a spill. That's what we are trying to avoid. Instead, if a parent could use words that paint the picture of the desired outcome, we might hear, "Be careful with your drink. Keep it all in the cup."

My last point is about neck pain. It's not just our words that create our reality; it's our thoughts, too. In the book *The Strangest Secret,* Earl Nightingale wrote, "We become what we think about." Words *and* thoughts are creative forces. In 1903, James Allen wrote in *As A Man Thinketh,* "All that a man achieves and all that he fails to achieve is the direct result of his own thoughts."

The lesson here is to be an observer of your words and your thoughts and use both wisely.

Geek alert: The British Medical Journal (BMJ) published data from the Global Burden of Diseases, Injuries and Risk Factors (2010), saying that neck pain is a serious public health problem. Some people live *for years* with neck pain. This same BMJ study ranks neck pain 4th highest on the list in terms of how many years people have lived with their neck pain.[12]

Neck pain inherently reveals a body out of balance. Certain energy imbalances correlate with certain aspects of biopsychosocial reasons for pain. The higher the degree of neck pain, the more attention needs to be given to the psycho-social distress of the client or patient.[13] What are examples of psycho-social stressors that affect everyday life?

Elevated work stress

Elevated home stress such as taking care of a family member (sick or healthy)

Regular exposure to hostility

A feeling of hopelessness, depression

Lack of job control

These stressors can manifest as neck pain. If you can alleviate the psycho-social factors, you can potentially alleviate the neck pain.

A cartoon image from Condé Nast shows this well visually. The man sitting in the oversized snow globe is a metaphor that he is protected from all the negativity surrounding him. Could you imagine yourself in a snow globe? You could feel separated from anybody who is a pain in the neck.[14]

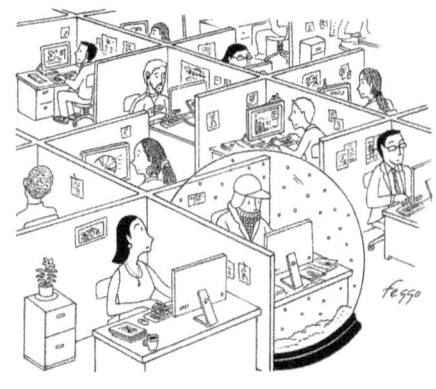

⌒ The Exercise ⌒

Now that we have changed the words we use and reframed the situation, we have one simple exercise to help contain and control your pain in the neck.

1. Identify who you think is the pain in the neck right now.
2. Take just a moment and bless them for who they are and how they show up on the planet.
3. Consider if the person is worth learning how to navigate in your life. Ask yourself: *Do they stay or do they go.*

If they stay:

a. Imagine the next encounter. Watch as if it were a movie or somebody else's encounter.
b. Imagine yourself in a large glass snow globe. There is a fresh air supply, so you can breathe easily. You can see and hear, but no negative vibrations can penetrate the

glass. Flowers, birds, the sun, and the moon gently float by when you speak.

c. Imagine the pain-in-the-neck person in a different snow globe. When they speak, bats, broomsticks, and skeletons float around. Maybe it's a Wizard of Oz snow globe, and there is a witch, some ruby red shoes, dirt, dust, and a big ol' house that could land on the person. There is so much debris that it's almost hard to see them. Make the snow globe any theme you want. See it in your mind's eye. They are in there. All their nonsense stays in there with them.

Are you worried about being a pain in the neck to someone else? I have listened to many of my clients who are too proud to ask for help. Pretending to be 'just fine.' Please consider making space in your life for the blessing that is *joyfully receiving*.

Hey, I get it. In the past, maybe *you* were always the one lending a hand. Now maybe you need a hand. It's a little harder to be the one eating at the soup kitchen than the one serving at the soup kitchen. Families who donated to the food pantry now need to shop at the food pantry. Be careful not to push away blessings by saying no. When a blessing shows up on your doorstep, do you deny it by saying, "Give that to someone else." Or "Others need it more than me." I've witnessed a person respond to praise and accolades, saying, "Not me. Oh, I don't deserve that."

How would it feel to just say thank you? Whisper those two words now. Say, "Thank you."

By mastering the humility it takes to say thank you, you will one day be back in the seat as a giver. If you are at a time in your life where you get to receive, celebrate. Breathe. Yes, it can be uncomfortable. Know that the Universe is teaching you the beautiful lesson of how to graciously receive. The universe is a world of balance. The Law of Giving and Receiving demonstrates the energetic flow back and forth. *If you block one part, you block the flow.* We get the full benefit when we happily give and receive in balance. And balance is what we need to relieve neck pain.

The snow globe visualization represents boundaries. That person who irritates you most likely crosses some boundaries. Or perhaps they have a chaotic lifestyle or see life completely differently than you do. This does not make either of you right or wrong. Putting people in the snow globe protects you. It also lets you off the hook. You don't need to help or be affected by their words or actions. You can say, "Not my monkey, not my circus."

After this little exercise, you can reward yourself! Rewards are essential for feeling encouragement and creating some momentum. What's your reward? A walk outside? A steamy bath? A warm cup of tea?

Today, we can thank that pain-in-the-neck for the lesson about boundaries and using our words intentionally.

See ya later, alligator.
Sending you much love and wishes for much relief.

Namaste,

Jodi

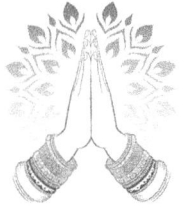

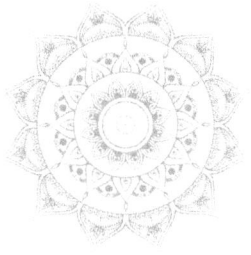

CHAPTER 3

HEADACHES

*I don't go by the rule book... I lead from
the heart, not the head.*

~ Princess Diana

Here Comes the Rain - Jennifer

Jennifer was with her dedicated daily chaperone and driver, Christine, one sunny summer morning. Jen was born with several special needs, and Christine supported Jen during the day – driving her to classes, doctor's office visits, making meals, monitoring meds, you name it. Christine laughs easily and had just the right balance of respect for Jen as a special needs adult and an old-school, take no bullshit attitude.

The two had a full day. They had just left water aerobics and were making a quick stop at Dunkin' Donuts for a little nourishment. Soon they would be off to pottery class.

Jen looked at the clear sky and projected, "Looks like rain." Christine thought Jen might have been trying to make an excuse to get out of going to class. But by the time Jen had her blueberry muffin in hand and they walked back to the car, a chilly breeze blew, and the sky was dark.

Jen looked at Christine and said, "Called it."

Jennifer could feel the weather changing. In her 30's, she started having what she called tsunami headaches. They would often come when a storm was rolling in, and the barometric pressure changed.

Like so many other days, Christine would call and reschedule class. Jen would get home just in time to crawl into bed before she started feeling nauseous. A few hours later, she would emerge from her dimly lit bedroom, ready to roll again.

I've never had a tsunami headache, but I have felt the wave of despair watching Jennifer curl up into a ball, barely able to respond to offers to help.

Jennifer was my sister.

To some degree I've hardened myself to hopeless feelings, opting instead to stay in faith. Holding the vision, saying a prayer, fingers crossed that "This too shall pass."

Headaches interrupt so many of the good times in life. Headaches have been directly linked to experiencing higher-than-normal levels of stress. Stress is a mental state of mind that produces physical symptoms. Stress can create a heightened emotional state. Emotional stress can lead to the physical symptoms of a headache or migraine.

Sometimes, headaches are caused by a misfunction of a person's biology. For example, low blood sugar, being overly tired, and eye strain are all physical reasons for a headache. Sometimes headaches are caused by invisible forces that overload stress onto our mental or emotional state of mind. Headaches are often a combination of all three conditions: physical, mental, and emotional.

What kind of stress causes a headache? Louise Hay said headaches can come from the pressure of wanting to be perfect. The rigid mindset of perfectionism. When we aren't perfect, that manifests as self-criticism.

Migraine headaches could be about resisting the flow of life or feeling that outside forces are controlling/driving your destiny.

Do either of those points of view resonate with you?

Jennifer wasn't a perfectionist; far from it. But, many outside forces impacted her day-to-day life. Due to complications of her rare condition, she had weekly medical appointments and frequent unpredictable trips to the Emergency Room. She regularly traveled for over an hour to see specialists. These external events were necessary, to be sure, but did they create an overabundance of emotional stress? Certainly.

However, Jennifer became very well-versed in communicating with psychologists, ER doctors, cardiac nurses, anesthesiologists, and others both in and out of a hospital setting.

One day, prepping for a heart catheterization, my mom and I sat with Jennifer as the anesthesiologist checked her blood oxygen levels. Jennifer was often her best advocate. That day, she pro-actively warned him, "Hey, don't freak out. My blood oxygen is going to be in the 80s." That was a normal level for Jen. He shot a glance at both my mom and me. We tried to look serious, but I cracked a smile, feeling proud of my little sister. My mom confirmed with a nod.

Jen's condition, Velocardiofacial Syndrome (VCFS), meant that quite a bit of blue blood circulated through her body.

Complications of a congenital heart defect, deoxygenated blood made its way back into her circulatory system. Yet another reason for her headaches.

Outsiders could stress her out, but my sister's headaches changed over the years.

At first, they coincided with her menstrual cycle. Doctors said hormones were the cause.

Then, a lifetime of low blood oxygen seemed to have an impact. Her blood got thicker. Doctors said this caused her headaches.

Her headaches could have been withdrawal symptoms as the pain medication dosage was cut back. Her medicine had gradually gotten stronger and stronger.

Jen's headaches would still come and go. Too often, the headaches would come and stay. For days. It was a torturous time for her and for those who loved her. It was a bumpy, emotional time.

Sometimes, underlying stress causes headaches. Sometimes, there's a straight-up biological reason for the pain. Jennifer had both and more.

No one had ever lasted over 30 years with the congenital heart defect known as Velocardiofacial Syndrome. That gave her a unique biology that was quite unprecedented and unpredictable. When Jen was born in 1977, doctors didn't know how to fix this heart defect. Now, they fix it in the first six months of life.

Jennifer wrapped up her work on this planet on the morning of March 4, 2015. She passed away peacefully in her sleep a few days before her 38th birthday. While it was difficult to say goodbye, I am at peace with her transition, knowing she is now in perfect health and happy.

Causes of Headaches

The causes of headaches are vast. Primary headaches like migraines and tension headaches come from chemical activity in the brain. Secondary headaches have specific causes, like sinus infection, pollution, or dehydration. Some people have a genetic predisposition to get headaches.

Almost all headaches are made worse by harsh environmental factors. Harsh environments are not limited to smog and pollen. According to the Mayo Clinic, "Anxious/stressful feelings are one of the most common headache triggers."[15] A harsh emotional environment can trigger a headache.

Many studies point to the fact that more anxiety or stress can increase headache pain intensity, while reduced anxiety can reduce headache pain intensity. This rationale makes sense, but do we put it into practice? Heightened levels of anxiety indicate a disconnect from the present. How do we decrease stress? We take a 'timeout' in life and bear witness to our state of mind. By giving ourselves a timeout, we disconnect from the external source of our stress. We have the opportunity to observe our state of being. When we observe our state, we become present.

In his book, *The Power of Now*, Eckhart Tolle summarizes the importance of being in the present moment by explaining that anxiety lives in the future.[16] Regret and resentment both only exist in the past. When experiencing a heightened level of anxiety, can you pause and observe your state? When you do, ask, "Am I in the past, present or future?" By coming back to the present, you will become aware that all is well in the present moment. In fact, you may want to say that out loud, "All is well in the present moment."

Geek Alert: Nature or Nurture? Biology or Biography?

In 1940 the Jim Twins, Jim Springer and Jim Lewis, were twins who were separated at birth. Through a series of wild circumstances, they eventually found each other and discovered astonishing similarities, including terrible headaches. They were tested and written about extensively. They shared identical DNA but grew up in very different lifestyles and circumstances. Yet, "Springer and Lewis both have peculiar elements to their headaches," said Dr. Leonard Heston, a member of the Minnesota research team. "The syndrome began at age 18 for both; each gets it with the same degree of disability and the same frequency — and they used almost identical words to describe it."[17]

They are biological brothers but grew up separately.

Heston isn't the only researcher connecting socio/environmental causes with biology. "Dealing with stress may be far more biological than we in the field have realized," said Dr. Joel R. Saper, director of the Michigan Headache and Neurological Institute in Ann Arbor. After learning about the twins' headaches, he wondered, "We may be dealing with biological programming here. That is, people may be born with a code that gives them a tendency to respond in a certain way to external or environmental factors. These twins may have opened up a fascinating new avenue."[18]

The research continues to help understand the origin of headaches. If you experience head pain, consider areas of your life that create stress. Are you holding any resentment or regret? The pain in your head could be a message to sort through these unresolved, mentally stressful memories.

When I catch myself feeling regret, I use my breath to come back to the current moment. I wiggle my toes. I ask my body, what does my body need right now? For me, it's usually some form of quiet, simple self-care. Cool water, warm coffee, to have a sit and think.

Coming back to the current moment, the present, reminds me that everything is okay right now.

Lesson: Improve Our Internal Dialogue

Words are important. In his famous book *The Strangest Secret*, Earl Nightingale teaches, "We become what we think about." Our internal conversation, also called self-talk, is massively important to our healing journey. Is your self-talk positive or negative? Do you call yourself an idiot? Do you tell yourself that you're so stupid? Hold, please. Would you call a friend an idiot? Would you tell a friend they are so stupid? I'm guessing you wouldn't speak to another human being the way you sometimes talk to yourself.

Let's consider energy, sound, and vibration. Did you know that some deaf people can 'hear' the piano playing by placing their hands on the outside of the instrument? As Beethoven lost his hearing, it is written that he would hold a wooden rod between his teeth to feel the music. To feel the *vibration* of the music. Music creates a vibration that can be absorbed by the body just like it's heard by the ears. If you've ever been to a rock concert, you may have left the building feeling like you were vibrating.

Words also create a vibration. Words have a vibe. When someone you love is upset, before they tell you, you can hear it in their voice. You can feel it in their words. You can feel it in the energy of the words. Positive and negative, our bodies absorb that vibration, that energy. What feeling do you want to create with your words? What vibration are you creating within your own body?

Is it the vibe of, "What's wrong with me?!"

Could the vibe shift to, "Hey, I look good!"

One other thought. How do you talk to little children? You may bend over. You may smile. You use compassion. You have patience. With little ones, we use words of encouragement versus criticism. How would it feel to talk to yourself like a child? Could you use compassion, patience, encouragement, and love in your internal dialogue?

Whether headaches are nature or nurture, science proves that when a person makes room to be more kind to themselves, their anxiety levels decrease. When you decrease the level of stress from a 9 to a 3, you proportionately decrease the pain level of a headache.

⌒ The Exercise: Breathwork ⌒

Since the cause of headaches can be internal and external, we will do a brief exercise that addresses both.

The "4-4-4" breathing pattern is a simple, straightforward tool to put in your toolbox. Just like it sounds, breathe in to the count of 4, hold the breath for the count of 4, breathe out for the count of 4. It is sometimes called a box breath.

> Step 1. Breathe in the cool, clear air for the count of 1, 2, 3, 4.
>
> Step 2. Hold the breath in. Count: 1, 2, 3, 4.
>
> Step 3. Exhale the breath to the count, 1, 2, 3, 4.
>
> Pause and check in with your body.

Repeat the 4-4-4 box breath one more time. Breathe in through the nose, 1, 2, 3, 4. Hold 2, 3, 4. Exhale 2, 3, 4. Tune into your body. What do you notice?

You can repeat this exercise whenever any part of your body feels heavy, sad, lonely, or angry. You can breathe the emotion out.

By breathing in a cool, clear breath and breathing out heavy emotions and feelings, we invite our body to release that which no longer serves us. By breathing in fresh air, we fill our lungs and bloodstream with fresh oxygen. Physiologically, additional oxygen helps to alleviate headaches.

We may not even know what old patterns or sadness might be stored, hidden, tucked away inside our mind and body. We can just offer an open invitation to release.

As you release the energy of the heaviness, the sadness, the depression - the *yuck* (we can just call it all *yuck*). As you release the yuck feeling, you make space for joy, for happiness. Even if the joy isn't immediate, a neutral feeling of contentment and/or peace will fill the space once occupied by the yuck.

Use this 4-4-4 breath anytime there is a feeling in your body you'd like to release. Coming back to the present moment, filling your lungs with fresh oxygen can decrease both the physical and psychological causes of headaches.

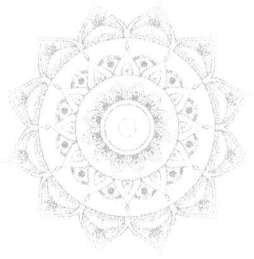

CHAPTER 4

THE THYROID

We delight in the beauty of the butterfly, but we rarely
admit the changes it has gone through
to achieve that beauty.

~ Maya Angelou

Why am I so tired? - Sarah

Sarah climbed the stairs to her bedroom. Her legs complained with each step. She had gained weight over the last year since her teenage daughter was diagnosed with depression and felt the strain on her joints as she climbed the stairs. For her daughter, puberty led to mood swings, a probable eating disorder, and self-harming. Sarah noticed the changes but didn't understand the depth of it until she saw the cut marks on her daughter's arm. This shocked her out of her denial.

On her mind was her neighbor, who had lost her son to an accidental overdose. This motivated Sarah to get her daughter into treatment. But it also meant that she must dedicate a good portion of her week to tasks assisting her daughter. She became the shuttle bus for multiple doctor's visits each week.

One day, she grabbed a nap while the tutor was there helping her daughter. A nap would give her the energy to make dinner for her husband and the kids. She was always so tired these days. As she laid her head down on the pillow, she, again, was aware of her weight gain. Sarah felt that she was eating like a bird, with barely any time to sit down and have a real meal. Her inner critic kicked in. *What is wrong here? How can I be gaining weight?* Her intuition was tap, tap, tapping. She thought something was off, but there was no time to investigate.

The frequent verbal and physical confrontations with her daughter were difficult to handle alone. In her husband's opinion, their daughter would just grow out of it. But Sarah worried. In the quiet moments, she admitted she didn't know if any of the counseling was working. Her mind swirled, *Will this ever end?* Every day she would tell herself, *I'll just take this nap* to face the rest of her day and fulfill her duty as a mother. She would soldier on.

Finally, the fatigue and weight gain prompted her to see her doctor. Her blood tests confirmed a medical condition called hypothyroidism. The thyroid is a gland that lives in the throat, just below the Adam's apple. This butterfly-shaped organ controls many different functions in the body but is mostly known for metabolism and temperature regulation. Sarah's condition of hypothyroidism meant that her thyroid was working too slowly. It wasn't producing enough hormones. Biologically, hypothyroidism is considered an autoimmune disease. For the next two years, she suffered from fatigue, weight gain, restless sleep, and intolerance of the cold.

Little by little, Sarah began to prioritize her own health. She learned how to communicate her own needs. Taking baby steps, she grew the courage to speak her truth. As she listened to her emotions, she got more comfortable saying *no* and sticking to healthy boundaries. Little by little, her body felt better. Her daughter's moods stabilized, but her marriage ended under years of strain. She had never imagined living alone. But she would rather face this new normal than be in the self-described hellhole that was her life.

With the added stress of the divorce, Sarah decided to make an appointment to get some individual counseling. She knew she needed to talk out loud to someone. Her therapist skillfully awakened Sarah's awareness of all the successes Sarah had in her life. She had an advanced degree from a prestigious D.C. university. She headed a successful international company. She had raised two smart, talented children. Sarah started to feel her normal self again: a strong, confident woman who was highly capable. By the time she became my client, she was energetic as she faced her new future with optimism.

Lesson: Quiet Your Inner Critic

What causes hypothyroidism? Doctors often don't know for sure. Biologically, it's a simple malfunction. It could be a side effect from another medication or an after-effect from a medical procedure. But Dr. Stephania Sciamento shines a light saying, "In my 10 years of medical practice, 1 in 5 women I treated had thyroid dysfunction of some kind. Each woman had a slightly different case, different history, and varied blood results. However, what did every single one of them have in common? Their inner self-talk was merciless. Every. Single. Woman. Especially the empathic ones."[19] Inner self-talk is fundamental to our health. And, like those diagnosed in Sciamento's practice, Sarah's inner critic was relentless.

Sarah's inner critic had a favorite topic: her weight. The voice would say things like, *You are a big, fat loser. Nobody really likes you. Who would want to be friends with you? Only other losers. You are just one failure after another. A lifetime of failures.* She assessed the worthiness of her life almost every day, feeling ashamed of her appearance. She'd joke about it, but deep down, she felt frustrated, lost, and sad.

Are you faced with a condition of the thyroid? Are you not speaking up about what's on your mind? Do you feel voiceless? In some ancient traditions, the throat is known as the Center of Communication and Self-Expression. Anatomically, the thyroid is the gateway between the heart and the head. According to other spiritual writings, the throat is the voice of human emotions. Maybe that's why, during an emotional moment, some say, "I had a lump in my throat." Or when we feel a strong emotion, we say, "Wow, I was all choked up."

I have heard my clients ask, "What's the point of talking about it? Nothing is going to change." You might be right. The situation may not change just by talking about it, but what *will* change is the bottled-up tension in your body. Release the words. Release the stagnant air you've been holding inside.

～ The Exercises: Treating Both Slow and Fast ～

Exercise for Hypothyroidism - Slow Thyroid
Because of the location of the thyroid, this exercise concentrates on balancing emotions by finding your words. Speak the following sentences out loud.

1. I get to do what I want to do. It's my turn.
2. I get to make my own rules now.

3. I speak up for myself. I am respected.

4. I am so grateful to feel free. I am hopeful. I love myself.

Other ways to use your voice include singing, reading poetry out loud, even watching a game show, and answering questions out loud.

The Mirror Test Exercise

You can practice finding your voice with the mirror test. Look in the mirror eye to eye.

1. Say out loud: "I love you."

2. Repeat Step One.

3. Try saying it naked.

Exercise for Hyperthyroidism - Fast Thyroid

Let's look at the flip side. Sometimes, the thyroid works too fast, a condition called hyperthyroidism. What does hyperthyroidism represent? According to psychologists researching from a biopsychosocial perspective, hyperthyroidism means a strong emotional reaction to being left out. Could this be part of your condition?

Consider the following questions:

1. Do I feel angry when I feel disrespected?

2. Do I speak my mind or stay silent when I feel angry?

3. Do I speak my truth at the moment, or do I replay the conversation over and over again, wishing I had said something else?

4. Where have I been left out? How does that make me feel?

5. Do other people worry about making me angry? (Others tip-
toeing around you?)

Now, you have one more piece of the puzzle. But what to do?
Asking the five questions above is the beginning. For many
readers, just knowing that rage is involved in the condition of
hyperthyroidism will help soften the negative effects. Talk therapy
helps. Meditation is divine. Breathwork will get to it.

Special Note About Hyperthyroidism

Certainly, there are emotions associated with hyperthyroidism.
Numerous research articles speak to this. One excerpt from the
book *Psychosocial Factors in Patients with Thyroid Disease* by
Petra Mandincova says, "Most contemporary studies support
[the] hypothesis that stress affects [the] origination and clinical
course of Graves' disease. Stress influences [the] immune system
directly or indirectly through [the] nervous and endocrine
system."[20] For both hypo and hyperthyroidism, healing begins
with finding your voice. Using your voice to speak your truth.

Whether you are dealing with a hypo or hyperthyroid
condition, evaluate how traditional medicine and complementary
medicine could work together for you. In treating any serious
condition, it's important to remember we have the opportunity
to show compassion to our body in the process. You are not
broken. Your body is recovering right now. You are patient with
everybody else. Can you be patient with yourself?

Elenor Roosevelt, 1884-1962, Former First Lady of the United
States said, *"No one can make you feel inferior without your consent."*

You are perfect, just the way you are today.

Wishing you courage to take action.

An Introduction to Chakras

Chakras (sha-krahs) are energy centers in the body. Starting at the tailbone up to the crown of the head, chakras follow the colors of the rainbow: Red/tailbone, orange/lower abdomen, yellow/solar plexus, green/heart, sky blue/throat, indigo blue/third eye and purple/crown. The thyroid is located in the throat. This gives us the indicator that we can treat the corresponding chakra energy center to help balance the thyroid. In the case of hypothyroidism, we set the intention to increase the vibration. And vice versa, for hyperthyroidism, we set the intention to calm the energy center. One of my favorite complementary options to treat the thyroid is to fortify the (throat) 5th chakra.

All of the energy centers or chakras in the body are assigned a color. The color of the 5th chakra is called true blue. It's sky blue. That true blue color can support balancing the thyroid. How does that work? That's a question people have been asking for thousands of years. What we do know are the actions we can take to incorporate more of the color sky blue into our daily routine. For example, we can wear a piece of jewelry in the color of sky blue (turquoise, topaz), swim in the big blue ocean, or even pick foods with blue color to support balance in that energy center. Food items like butterfly pea flowers (herbal tea), blue crab, blue corn chips, and blue caviar. Since blue foods are limited, we could incorporate other choices into our routine that soothe the throat. Drinking herbal tea, using honey and lemon, drinking coconut water, and for added fun, consider adding Blue Curaçao blueberries to your beverage of choice.

It's easy to wear true blue gemstones like Swiss blue topaz or aquamarine. However, you may be more comfortable with an intentional clothing selection. Could you wear a blue tie? Have a blue pocket square? Could you wrap a blue pashmina around your shoulders? Wear a pair of sapphire cufflinks or a necklace, perhaps? This simple action is a nod to the Universe supporting your healing journey.

There are many other options in complementary medicine to support treating both hypo and hyperthyroid conditions. Integrative options include adding iodine to your weekly menu. (Low iodine is a major cause of hypothyroidism.)

To increase your natural intake of iodine, consider eating saltwater fish like cod, sea bass, or haddock 2 or 3 times a week. Grab a seaweed salad or enjoy a sushi roll wrapped in nori (black wrapper/dried seaweed), which will also add iodine to your system. Iodized salt is also readily available. If you are already taking thyroid medication, inform your doctor about any additional supplements or dietary changes.

Beyond diet, consider acupuncture, visiting a homeopathic doctor, or seeing an osteopathic doctor specializing in the condition. No appointment is necessary to do Contrast Hydrotherapy, a treatment you can do at home. Alternate heat and cold to the neck/throat area. Studies show this may stimulate thyroid functions. St. Luke's Hospital recommends 3 minutes heat to 1 minute cold and alternating 3 times for one set (12-15 minutes). For the best effect, do 2-3 sets per day.[21]

A Note About Crystals

Mary Ancillete, a spiritual teacher, therapist, and writer from the UK, taught me about crystals.[22] Some people have found relief for their thyroid problems using blue crystals. If you're a little shy about wearing big jewelry or being seen as a woo-woo person, just carry a few stones in your pocket. Having them on your body will give you the vibe of the stone.

Choose your crystal:

1. Aquamarine (Stone of Courage)
2. Angelite (Stone of Awareness)
3. Lapis Lazuli (Stone of Friendship, Truth/Total Awareness)
4. Blue Lace Agate (Stone of Articulation)
5. Blue Kyanite (High Vibration Stone)
6. Blue Apatite (Stone for Personal Power)
7. Turquoise (Stone of Communication)
8. Sodalite (Harmonizing Stone)
9. Azurite (Stone of Heaven)

I'm not here to convince you a pocket full of rocks will solve your thyroid issues. I am here to remind us we are all a bag of bones, water, and blood that is alive because of our *innate energy.* An energy that all living things have including trees, grasshoppers, and the ocean. We sense that energy. Carry a few blue stones in your purse or pocket. You can tell people it's for luck. If you choose to include stones or crystals in your life, let them breathe a little. They need some sunshine now and then. Like a plant, those stones absorb the energy from the sun and get even more positively infused when you thank them for their support.

As you find what works for you, you may be amazed at the shift in the ease of your communication. You'll feel proud of how calmly you know and speak your truth. For some, physical symptoms just seem to quietly go away when we address the underlying causes. This is an example of empowering yourself with tools available to help remedy some of the symptoms your body is experiencing.

If this seems a little out there, remember this is a philosophy, not a religion. This is a suggestion to explore what works for you, not an invitation to worship a false idol. Continue to pray. Continue to do your form of the church thing. A stone is not considered a false god. For me, it's a representation of the beauty of the planet. God gives us wonderful things on the planet to support us. Consider the gifts from Mother Earth: wood for fireplaces, trees to change CO_2 into fresh oxygen, shells that are jewels from the sea, beautiful gems, and crystals to strengthen our souls.

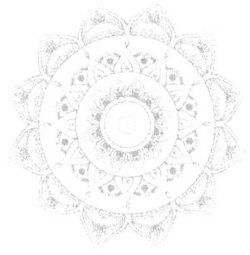

CHAPTER 5

THE SHOULDERS

The body keeps the score.

~ Dr. Bessel van der Kolk,
Neuroscientist

Weight of the World - Maria

During one of our many online video calls, Maria winced and touched her left shoulder. I asked, "Is your shoulder bothering you?" She nodded and said, "I think I slept on it wrong. What do you think?" Well, obviously, we were not in the same room. I couldn't physically touch her, so I was at a bit of a disadvantage. Maria had been helping me with social media, so she had become well versed in the message in the pain. Nevertheless, I asked, "Are you open to exploring the roots of your pain?" She agreed.

I gently reminded her that pain sometimes has its roots in mental or emotional stress. Shoulders represent responsibility.

Left shoulder pain could imply that there is an imbalance of responsibility in a traditionally feminine role. Feminine roles include being a mother, a grandmother, or a daughter. Domestic tasks like cooking, cleaning, and being the major caregiver to the kids have traditionally been considered feminine roles. I asked Maria if there was an imbalance in her life, a place she felt she had taken on too much responsibility.

Maria was silent while I spoke. Then her eyes opened wide, and she said, "Well, I don't know if this is related, but I'm a single mother."

At that moment, the message of her pain crystallized. Maria was taking on both the feminine and masculine roles of parenting. She had very little help. Her parents hadn't wanted her to keep the child. But Maria couldn't bear the idea of giving up her daughter. So, at 20, when most of her friends worried about which fraternity to visit or which early morning class to cut, she was working and a full-time parent. This created an imbalance.

The message her left shoulder wanted to share with her was that doing this all alone was too much. She didn't need to be a hero. She could look for help.

Maria looked like she had seen a ghost. "That's weird, she said." Her secret struggle wasn't really a secret. Maria decided it was time to get some outside help. With the help of a local community organization, she found specific services to help her as a single mom. Maria's shoulder pain eased up. She started dating a lovely young man who adored her and her baby girl. After what she called "a proper courtship," they married and had a second child. They continue to be devoted to each other and are raising their growing family.

As I identify the specific message in the painful parts of the body, it often seems like a strange coincidence, but chronic pain sends a clear message. Consider if your shoulder pain could represent responsibilities that are out of balance in your life.

Are My Parents Getting Old? - Stan

Stan was experiencing right shoulder pain. As an amateur triathlete, he had plenty of battle scars. As we discussed his pain, we determined it was highly unlikely he'd aggravated an old injury. He had only been doing half the training since his mom and dad moved in. One morning, he woke up out of the blue with sharp distracting shoulder pain.

If your pain is *out of the blue* it is a great time to explore the biopsychosocial connection. I asked Stan if we could explore any new mental or emotional stress in his life as it could contribute to the pain.

In his gentle southern accent, he explained his mom and dad had been living with him for the past three months. His parents were aging and required more attention than they were getting living independently. He and his wife agreed; the situation wasn't going to improve. The last time they went to a Major League Baseball game, his dad needed to take breaks on the walk from the handicapped parking spot to their seats. He no longer had the endurance, relying more heavily on his cane.

His mom, on the other hand, could lift her suitcase out of the trunk. But she had asked the same questions over and over again. And when it came time to make her world-famous oatmeal cookies, she was having trouble following the recipe. Stan and his wife had to change their lifestyle to accommodate his parents. But his parents also had to dramatically change their lifestyle, moving away from their lifelong home to move in with him and his wife. With four adults in the house, it was a period of adjustment for everyone.

Stan loved having them close, but he knew that their aging conditions would soon require more help. Stan started to research home health aids and assisted living homes, but his parents wanted nothing to do with it. They're from a generation of private folks. They had no interest in having a strange person helping them out of the shower. As a son, Stan wanted to respect his parents' requests. Knowing that at some point he may have had to defy his parents' wishes to get them the care they required meant he was living in constant conflict.

He said, "This is like trying to figure out how to put socks on a rooster." Despite his humor, he was in serious mental anguish about planning the future with/for his parents. Then his shoulder started acting up.

Once Stan described the situation at home, I could hear the message his shoulder pain was saying. Stan was feeling overburdened with this responsibility. We chatted about how he could share the responsibility of ensuring his parents are well taken care of. Could he ask his siblings to get involved? What were some realistic options, short-term and long-term?

A few weeks went by, and I saw Stan again. I asked about his shoulder pain. He chuckled and said, "Jodi, this is weird. My shoulder has been feeling much better. I have to admit; it started feeling better when my sister and I talked about Mom and Dad. She says she wants them to come live with her!" Stan's sister and her husband had already converted their garage into an in-law apartment, and they wanted Stan's parents to live with them. They even had daytime help lined up. I was surprised by how quickly he found a resolution. Or maybe I should say how quickly the universe sent the solution. Shrugging his not-sore shoulders, Stan smiled and said, "Yep, and Mom and Dad love the idea!"

Let's review this right shoulder pain pattern. The right side of the body represents masculine roles such as grandfather, father, and son. Traditionally, masculine tasks include acting as the head of a household, making money, and enjoying beer, cigars, and sports. Shoulders represent burdens or responsibilities. Stan's right shoulder pain may be sending a message about his mental stress. He saw the imbalances he was creating in his own life when he began taking on the role of caretaker of his parents. Yet he willingly took on the burden of responsibility as the son. Was it just a coincidence that his shoulder pain disappeared after finding a solution to the emotional dilemma?

The Lesson: Beast of Burden

What burden are you carrying more than your fair share of?

What chronic shoulder pain experience has taught me is that pain is trying to get our attention to make a change. Because shoulders represent balance, shoulder pain may require you to examine any imbalances in your life. Shoulders also carry weight, which can sometimes be seen as a burden. Consider the mule, sometimes called a beast of burden because it carries things on its back. Shoulder pain could mean that your burdens are too heavy, and you will need to let go of some of the emotional weight you have been carrying.

When we acknowledge the imbalance of the situation, we demonstrate that we are listening to our bodies. We are listening to the pain and translating the story. Think about the language you hear people saying, like the following phrases. *It feels like the weight of the world is on my shoulders. At work, I'm always looking over my shoulder. I've been putting my shoulder to the wheel on this project.* These sayings about the shoulder all represent a mindset of work and burden that can manifest as shoulder pain.

Part of the problem could be the mental and emotional stress of caretaking. Both of the stories about Maria and Stan had to do with taking on extra responsibilities as caretakers.

Even if the job is *just* getting the kids to school on time. Tasks like *just* getting your parents to the doctor or *just* taking down the holiday lights can feel like burdens when we feel there is no help. Or when there is no reward. It is then that our bodies will begin to nudge us as a reminder to slow down and do some self-care. When we reward ourselves, we are empowered. Studies prove that planned rewards keep us motivated and happy.

Shoulder pain normally takes 2-4 weeks to resolve physically and mentally. That's about the time it takes to recognize and figure out how to re-balance responsibilities, plan rewards, and potentially ask for help. Shoulder pain may be a physical overuse injury, but if you pay attention, it may be your invitation to acknowledge and release a burden you hadn't even considered.

⌒ The Exercise: Say Out Loud ⌒

Let's breathe. Take a slow, deep breath in as you count to four. Hold your breath for seven seconds. Breathe out for eight seconds.

If you're comfortable, do that again. It's called 4-7-8 breathing. Breathe out through your mouth. Maybe make a *hah* sound as you exhale. Imagine stress leaving your body as you *hah*. Feeling better?

Give yourself permission to *not know* how to solve the problem, but just recognize the challenge.

1. Say out loud, "I feel a burden when I think about _____."
   It could be a situation, a current issue, or a person.

2. Say out loud, "I take on more than my fair share of responsibility with _____."

3. Say out loud, "I feel a burden when _____."

In my experience, when you state the challenge exactly, the universe kicks into action to deliver a solution. It's wild when the solution is just so perfect that you couldn't have planned it better yourself.

I love the affirmation, "I am positively expecting great things no matter what I see before me. The universe is rearranging itself on my behalf right now!" And so it is.

Much love and light as you consider your balance of roles and responsibilities.

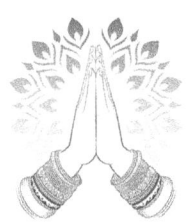

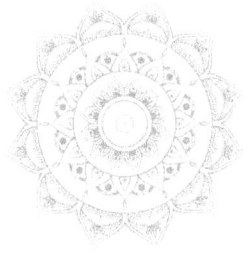

CHAPTER 6

THE LUNGS

*Sometimes it's okay if the only thing you did
today was breathe.*

~ Yumi Sakugawa

Unexpressed Grief - Marcy

Marcy chose to let her hair be its natural salt-n-pepper color. In the corporate world, being seen as aging can be a disadvantage, but she didn't care. A tennis aficionado and a lifelong competitor, she believed in getting massages on a regular schedule. As was standard in my practice, before her session I asked her, "How's your body feeling today?"

Never one for whining, Marcy revealed some new information. In a very matter-of-fact way, she told me she was getting bronchitis as she did every year when summer changed to fall. Marcy was 50+ years old with a textbook healthy lifestyle. She eats well, works out, and doesn't smoke. But every year, she gets bronchitis?

This piqued my interest. Before her next appointment, I did some research. I wanted to offer some options on how complementary medicine can support the lungs. At her next session, I went through my list of healthy options. To my surprise, she was already doing everything I mentioned. Omega 3 fatty acids, check. Breathe easy, check. Tea, check. Echinacea, Vitamin C, Eucalyptus oil, check, check, check. *Except* there was one piece of information that was new.

When I mentioned that lungs represent grief, she stared at me. I went on to say that Traditional Chinese Medicine teaches that lung afflictions speak to unexpressed grief. Marcy sat silently, staring through me. I could tell she was time-traveling back to a memory. I remained quiet, and it felt like a month before she spoke. Her voice cracked just a little when she said, "I guess that could apply. I've never really gotten over the death of my mother when I was 14."

I was stunned. In the two years I worked with her, she never mentioned her mom had passed. The massage session was pretty quiet that day as we both considered unexpressed grief and how it related to annual bronchitis.

Geek alert: Symptoms Are a Sign of Disharmony

German doctors and co-authors Dethlefsen and Dahlke, in their book *Healing Power of Illness: Understanding What Your Symptoms Are Telling You,* explain, "In short, disease is a state that indicates the individual, in his (or her) consciousness, has ceased to be in order or harmony. The loss of internal balance manifests itself in the body as a symptom. The symptom is, therefore, a signal and carrier of information, since with its appearance, it interrupts the rhythm of our life and forces us to be aware of it."[23]

Symptoms are a signal. A messenger. In this case, Marcy contracting bronchitis every year was the symptom, but also a signal. A sign that something was out of order or an inner knowing of the lack of harmony. The unexpressed emotion created disharmony. She never gave herself permission to explore and express the grief of losing her mom. There are a host of repercussions connected to Marcy's mom's death. She grew up too fast by having to act as the mother of the family. Her family didn't like drama, so she was expected to be strong and move on by ignoring her emotions. Her house was a quiet one where any outbursts were cause for discipline. Marcy had been unable to express natural grief with tears or even talk about how she felt. She was told that big girls don't cry. Had she been permitted to cry, her tears would have allowed her to empty out the pain she sequestered inside her lungs. In time, expressed emotion can lead to naturally re-living happy memories and can help reclaim the feeling of joy.

Marcy decided to do some talk therapy and breath work that fall. After starting her protocol, winter arrived. And for the first time since her mother's death, she did not get bronchitis.

Using Busy Work as a Distraction - Ellie

Recently, my friend Ellie lost both her mother and father within four months of each other. She'd barely gotten through the funeral for her mom when her dad ended up in hospice care. Even though her dad said he was ready to go, Ellie wasn't ready for him to go. She was still processing the sadness of her mom's death when she had to spring into action to be there for her dad. When we talked, she could only say, "Sometimes that's how life goes."

The weekend came, and Ellie was packing the car, ready to head off to the nursing home to see her dad when she received a call. The nursing home had just gone on strict lockdown. No visitors. The COVID pandemic was in its early stages and was known to infect vulnerable populations, especially frail residents in nursing homes. A decision had been made - only essential staff were let in or out. No visitors. Ellie's dad passed away just a few days later. She knew it was coming, but still, she could barely breathe.

Although they had spoken on the phone several times, and she knew her dad had said he was ready, Ellie didn't get a chance to see him that one last time. She didn't get to give him one more hug. She didn't really say goodbye. She felt like the wind had been knocked out of her.

As late summer turned to fall, Ellie still felt wounded. On any given day, all her activities were related to settling her parents' estate: sending copies of death certificates, returning calls from lawyers, notarizing documents, dealing with insurance and banks, and getting valuations of the assets. She was busy with important tasks and in turn buried much of her sadness.

Even in the tornado of activity, she knew something was off. Normally, she could work like a horse. Now, she struggled to stay healthy. Recently, a respiratory infection turned into pneumonia. She purposefully stayed isolated. But her weakened condition concerned her family. A good friend, who is also an Acupuncturist, came to visit. That afternoon, over tea, she pointed out that the lungs are associated with repressed grief. The lungs can become vulnerable to infection when we put on the strong front, sporting a stiff upper lip.

Ellie finally put two and two together when a final electric bill arrived a few days later. Out of the blue, she was weeping.

Intellectually, she couldn't understand why she would fall to pieces over such an innocuous piece of mail. It was a tipping point. The accumulation of bottling up the emotions and her friend's gentle reminder, led Ellie to tap into her emotions. She felt her tears were completely irrational. I assured her they were 100% rational and necessary.

Ellie decided to start mourning the death of her parents and the subsequent selling of her childhood home by creating social media posts honoring her mom and dad's lives. She began to breathe easier. She started doing Pranayama breathwork classes to strengthen her lungs, a practice she continues today. During yoga, when the instructor says, "Take a deep breath," Ellie is grateful every time she can do so.

It is healthy to be sad whenever that feeling arrives. Sadness can be triggered by a song, a smell, a face that looks so familiar. Feel the feeling. So often, we put on a brave face instead of allowing and exploring the feeling. It's healthy to mourn, even if that sadness comes at a time that's not convenient. Your life will continue in between the waves of sadness. Give yourself permission to mourn. It's not weak. It's one of the bravest things you can do for yourself. As you become more comfortable expressing and releasing grief, you will find that it helps your lungs get stronger, too.

The Lesson: Lungs Represent Unexpressed Grief

For about 2000 years, Traditional Chinese Medicine (TCM) has taught that lung distress represents unexpressed grief. Western medicine does not share this belief. Western medicine has its roots in chemistry. As of this writing, scientists have identified about 118 elements in the *chemical world*. A little over 150 years ago, chemists Mendeleev and Meyer created early versions of the Periodic Table. Western medicine leans on pharmaceutical interventions to help a body heal.

Western medicine has benefited greatly from chemistry and interpretation of elements and compounds. The world population lives longer because of life-saving drugs, vaccines that eradicate disease, and a deeper understanding of the physical composition of things.

But Traditional Chinese Medicine took the elements a step further. TCM focuses on the Five Elements of the *material world*. These elements are fire, earth, water, wood, and metal. One important consideration to assess a condition from this point of view, we need to understand that these descriptions are not literal.

A brief explanation is appropriate. When we think about wood, we think of a tree. A tree is strong and flexible. Trees grow and make steady progress. Wood is natural and warm. This is the identity of wood.

Likewise, the element of water is not literally water. It is the characteristics of water. Water flows. Water can be deep, quiet. This is the energy of water.

The Earth element represents the energy of nurturing and gives life.

The characteristics of metal are strong, firm, and structured.

And fire burns hot. It clears the way. It's intense, warm, and happy.

As in chemistry, TCM combines elements. Most people are a combination of primarily two of these five elements. One thing both theories (Eastern and Western) are clear about is that a healthy body operates with balance in each element. A healthy body operates at its best when it isn't too cold or hot, or too wet or dry. Too much of any element creates an imbalance. Too much water puts out fire. Too much fire burns wood and melts metal. In treating a physical condition, it is helpful to understand both traditional and western points of view. Wet lungs can create an environment that fosters infection. Dry lungs imply constrained or restricted airways that may be attached to emotions.

In the real world, we see real life examples. In the construction world, workers get exposed to asbestos but some don't get sick. Tens of thousands of people smoke and never get lung cancer. *So why are your lungs a challenge?* Could it be buried grief?

At times the external environment creates irritation of the lungs, including factors like allergies and pollution. Other times I have been told, "Since I was a kid, I've always had issues with my lungs." In my opinion, no child has had the chance to accumulate enough unexpressed grief to give themselves a lung condition. Yes, it could be an allergy or a genetic predisposition. Consider, what if that little one was born with sadness? Are you the parent of one of those old soul kids? Not all of those old souls struggle to breathe, but some do. Maybe *you were one* of those kids.

Here's a stretching moment: Would you consider hypnosis to discover a past life?

Hypnotherapy

If you have had issues with your lungs since you were a child, it could indicate a past life challenge. Whether you believe in past lives or not, what if? What if your discovery resolved your lung issues?

In the book, *Many Lives Many Masters,* author Dr. Brian Weiss shares his experience as a psychotherapist. He tells the story of treating a female client who had recurring nightmares and paralyzing fear from extreme anxiety.

Dr. Weiss, as he had done many times before, uses hypnotherapy to bring his patient back to her earliest memory of fear. What shocked them both was that the client clearly recalled a past life. The trouble was, Dr. Weiss didn't believe in past lives. At least he didn't at that time. Nonetheless, after the session, his patient reported no more anxiety.

The next visit produced more progress. His skepticism evaporated as this unexpected and amazing success story unfolded. Past life regression proves to be an effective and beneficial tool many qualified psychotherapists use to help their clients discover the unknown past, which in turn assists in overcoming their symptoms.

Dr. Weiss wrote about his concern regarding sharing this new and unusual experience with colleagues. He was worried he would completely discredit himself as a doctor. But he gained credibility. When you shine a light, darkness disappears and lights the way for others to follow.

For many people, chronic lung problems include a connection to unexpressed grief. Lungs represent sadness, not breathing in the joy of life. Control is also a major part of respiratory illnesses. Being controlled by someone else or someone's expectations quite literally can suck the wind out of you.

Unexpressed grief indicates the tears that were never cried. It is the sadness never expressed, buried in your chest - not coincidentally in close proximity to your heart. It's the imaginary neat little box sealed tightly where all those emotions are stored. The box holds the story of our pain and is a good indicator of where we may be ready to heal now. When you are willing to peek under the lid, gently ask yourself to acknowledge that there might be something there. It's in the denying or ignoring of the emotions that affliction persists. Not being able to breathe comfortably affects every other part of your life. Be curious. Explore if it relates to some old sadness. That's when the healing begins.

Perhaps a past life is a bit too far for you, but accessing a past *moment* you haven't given thought to can open a door to understanding.

How Do You Deal with Sadness?

Melanie Creedy, Australian Registered Homeopath (AROH), warns in her blog[24] *Symbolism of Illness, the Lungs & Breath*, "Suppression of asthma [or any condition] with conventional medication pushes the symptoms ever deeper, denying us the opportunity to resolve issues which may go back years and even generations. Perhaps the question to ask is, 'How much do I really want to release myself from restriction and be able to enjoy and breathe in life?'"

If you have been dealing with lung issues, consider asking, *What sadness have I not fully mourned?* It's healthy to be sad.

Can you sit with sadness and give it a voice? Or does it seem easier to swallow it and stay busy? Some believe it's more comfortable and convenient to avoid the messiness of sadness. They pass on funerals, avoid sending condolence cards, and wait a while before calling anyone who has lost a loved one, characterizing it as embarrassing or uncomfortable. Maybe, but for whom?

Have you been through a big loss? Did you self-isolate? If you normally freeze, not wanting to talk about sadness, I encourage you to make space for sadness and pain. How do we make space to feel some feelings? A key question is, are you ready to feel some feelings? If you can say, "I'm ready," one way to make space is to invite a close friend to share a cup of tea. Creating a safe environment could be enough. You don't have to say anything. Set the intention that you will begin the process just by being in a safe place with someone you trust. Then, *if you want to*, you could talk about it. You may be ready gently and slowly to open just a little.

Grief can come in some unexpected situations. It might be the loss of a pet, the end of a job, the end of a relationship, or even moving from a home. These events may be anticipated or even planned, but the timing of feeling grief is unpredictable.

You know the date you will retire from work or your last day in the house where you raised your kids, yet the sentimental feelings of a life well-lived can wash over you. These life events may be for the highest good of all concerned, but it can still be sad. You have permission to feel sad.

⌇ The Exercise: Feeling Your Emotions ⌇

Sit in a safe and comfortable space with a pen and paper. This exercise will need to be repeated daily or weekly for as long as you experience lung discomfort.

1. Breathe in slowly through your nose.

2. Exhale slowly through your mouth making a *sssssssss* sound. Repeat this pattern three times.

3. Without overthinking, write a list of things, people, or situations you have lost in your life.

4. Repeat the inhale and exhale with your eyes closed.

5. Keeping your eyes closed, pay attention to your body. Where does it feel restricted? What aches? Imagine breathing oxygen in and sending it directly to those parts of your body.

6. Now, write any emotions you feel when you consider the items on your list.

7. Allow yourself time to sit with the emotions.

With each item, breathe in deeply, filling your lungs and belly with air. As you exhale, imagine releasing the sorrow through your mouth. In your exhale, allow your vocal cords to make a noise to acknowledge the pain and its release.

Decoding the reasons for a chronic lung condition takes more than just understanding the biology. It takes an understanding of the mental and emotional stressors that may be quietly affecting our bodies. Unexpressed grief can cause a level of consistent low-grade sadness, bouts of depression, and a tendency toward self-isolation. Containment of those emotions may cause a restriction within your lungs. To inhale and fill the lungs with healthy oxygen, grief and loss must be exhaled. A teacher of groundbreaking breathing techniques and TEDx speaker, Max Strom, says, "Some doors only open from the inside."[25] Meaning that sometimes, we don't heal from the outside in; we have to heal from the inside out.

Peace to you on your journey. You are brave. You are safe.

All is well, really.

Hugs.

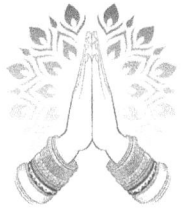

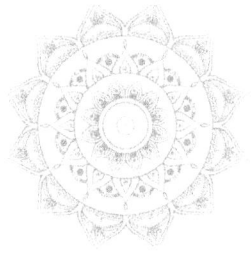

CHAPTER 7

THE WRISTS

*Life is really simple, but we insist on making
it complicated.*

~ Confucius

Tunnel Vision - Tina

Tina came to me with wrist pain. She worked as a high-powered executive assistant to the president of a large global organization. She booked all his travel and hotels. She organized his calendar. She managed his emails.

As the years went by, he relied more and more on Tina outside of normal working hours. She was single, so she didn't mind the extra work. Tina was a model employee in the eyes of her boss and the company. She was a tall, confident woman who worked with a vibrant brilliance. Her job required her to be on her computer for hours and hours every day. The cause of her wrist pain certainly was related to repetitive stress.

But as you have no doubt guessed, there was more to the story. She was starting to get frustrated with her ever-expanding job duties. Her work life bled into her personal life. She was effectively always on call. Tina did a beautiful job managing his work/life balance. Until the life side began to grate on her. Originally, she thought it a sign of trust when he asked her to use her great taste to pick out a gift for his wife for their anniversary, but he never thanked her.

She told herself it was okay. He was very generous. Often, he'd give her gift cards to get her nails done or to a hot new restaurant. And her bonuses were not insignificant. Unfortunately for Tina, his monetary attention started to feel inauthentic. In her opinion, he needed to do some of his own personal stuff. And she needed to have off hours that were dedicated solely to herself that he could not breach. All too often, a random text message would show up at 10:00 pm asking, "What time is my flight tomorrow?"

Tina knew she had put herself in this situation. She was the one who made herself indispensable. Now, she couldn't get as much done because of her wrist pain. Tina couldn't pick up the teapot or pour milk into her cup. She dropped things regularly. Her condition was severe enough that her doctor told her she needed to schedule carpal tunnel surgery. It was the only way to relieve the throbbing pain.

Tina didn't want to get surgery. Her gut was saying there must be other options. In the past, she turned to massage therapy for some neck pain and found the treatment provided her with great relief. She was optimistic an orthopedic massage therapist would be able to advise her. To her, surgery seemed too extreme.

Tina was my first client with a serious case of Carpal Tunnel Syndrome. The physical nerve pathway between the neck and the wrist impacts the condition. I wasn't surprised to determine that

Tina's mental stress contributed to this condition. During her sessions, we discovered the underlying reasons Tina's wrists were screaming at her. In this case of Carpal Tunnel Syndrome, the physical relief was almost immediate after the massage. She was pain-free for three days. But the condition would consistently return until she addressed all the reasons for the pain.

Tina seemed to have it all: cool apartment, fancy car, fashionable purses, elegant shoes. She fed her soul by volunteering at the local no-kill Animal Shelter. She had a great relationship with her family and often had Sunday dinners together. However, in the midst of it, she was losing some important parts of who she was as an individual.

She used to love going to the gym, but now, with the imbalance in her life, she was lucky if she made it twice a week. Additionally, she was exhausted from working a job that had become her whole life.

Eventually, Tina explained to her truly considerate boss that she was working too much. The workload had increased over the years. Her body had indicated that it was time for an additional assistant. Tina knew her job couldn't last forever, especially at her pay rate. She was at the top of the pay scale. She asked herself, "What do I want the future to look like?"

Tina happily trained a new hire to help take some of the work off her plate. Fortunately, her boss was pulling back as well. He stopped accepting so many invitations to travel. Just 12 months later, the company sold, and Tina moved into a new role. Her new role had much less responsibility and less visibility within the company. She was thrilled with her new position. She had 'wished' this new role into being. She enjoyed more free time and got back to the gym. Later that year, she met the man who was to become her husband. The future she imagined gradually came to pass. Is it possible that her wrist not only sent her a message but created the gap that her mind and body needed to move forward?

The Lesson: Wave Goodbye

I love wrist pain. Let me clarify, I love to work on wrists to help alleviate the pain. Wrists respond really well to massage therapy, physical therapy, heat/ice, and other physical treatments. When wrist pain is present, we get the opportunity to ask *why* the pain showed up. Was there a specific event that triggered your wrist pain? An ambitious pose in yoga class? A fall on the ice? Twelve hours of typing? Or is this pain *out of the blue*?

Wrists represent flexibility. Consider what the wrist does.

The wrist moves the hand. What movements does the wrist make? Healthy wrists can move the hand down and up. The wrists will move the thumb toward the body and the pinky finger away from the body in a waving motion. They wave. Since flexibility is its normal state, wrist pain can indicate being inflexible. Not physically inflexible. *Mentally or emotionally* inflexible.

Not everyone who has wrist pain faces flexibility issues. Sometimes, the pain is simply median nerve impingement due to wrist compartment compression. The wrist is an incredible structure. It's made up of eight carpal bones that form a bridge/an arch. I think of the carpal tunnel like the stone arches that form a bridge over a river. The back of the wrist is the top of the arch. The wrist on the palm side is where the Transverse Carpal Ligament lives. Imagine a watch strap wrapped around your wrist. That is similar to the Transverse Carpal Ligament. This ligament stabilizes the wrist and helps hold the carpal bones in place.

When things are flowing smoothly, there is plenty of room for the nerves, tendons, bones, blood, etc. However, typing on a keyboard can compress that area. Long spans of time with the wrist bent can compromise the median nerve that runs through this tunnel. Over days, weeks, and months, the part of the wrist that faces the desk gets compressed, and the nerves become irritated. Sometimes, the bones move, but mostly, it's the Transverse Carpal Ligament—the watchband area—that shortens and tightens.

In Western medicine, the protocol is predictable. Step 1: anti-inflammatory medicine. If that doesn't work, Step 2: splinting. Still in pain? Step 3: surgery.

A Word about Carpal Tunnel Surgery

Around 1854, doctors started using a neutral splint to alleviate symptoms of Carpal Tunnel Syndrome. That technique is still used today. Around 1924, a surgeon decided the act of cutting the tendon would be a good option to relieve the pressure. If you were wearing a watch and it was too tight on your wrist, what would you do? Loosen it, right? Yes. To me, cutting the watch off your wrist seems a little extreme. Yet, that's basically what happens in carpal tunnel release surgery.

The Transverse Ligament is severed to release the pressure that has built up in the Carpal Tunnel. Instant relief for the patient. No more pressure. Lots of physical therapy, but no more pain, right? Not always. Sometimes, when that ligament heals, it gets thick with scar tissue. The thick scar tissue can take up more than the normal amount of space in the Carpal Tunnel. As a result, scar tissue can build up, putting pressure on the nerves, bones, blood vessels, etc. The solution becomes the problem.

When my new client, Lily, arrived, I noticed a nasty scar on her wrist. At first, I approached cautiously. The incision at the heel of her hand was about 3" long. It was the first time I had seen someone healing from carpal tunnel surgery. It looked very invasive and painful. Lily assured me her wrist pain was gone, but now she was getting massage specifically in this area to regain full range of motion, hopefully decrease the build-up of scar tissue, and proactively minimize the risk of any problems with the other wrist.

This case is why I am a big fan of working on wrists. When I learned what Lily and other clients had been through (daily throbbing pain, surgery, PT/recovery), I wanted to help prevent/reverse this condition if at all possible.

In the non-judgmental space of the massage treatment room, Tina felt safe to share. When telling your story out loud to another person, sometimes it comes out differently. In explaining your story, you may see it from a different point of view.

By saying your truth out loud: *I'm working too much. I'm feeling stressed. It's a lot of pressure to keep juggling all the balls in the air.* Or *I don't want to keep feeling like this*, you hear yourself telling your truth. You have articulated the problem more clearly. You named the elephant in the room. Then, healing begins from within.

⌒ Exercise: Being Flexible ⌒

Grab a pen. Ask yourself:

1. In what situation could you be more flexible?
2. What do you want to wave hello to?
3. What do you want to wave goodbye to?

As you answer these questions in your head, formulate a sentence.

I could be more flexible with _____.

I welcome and wave hello to _____.

It is time for me to wave goodbye to _____.

Whisper the sentence out loud.

I could be more flexible with _____.
I am waving hello to _____.
I am waving goodbye to _____.

What baby step could you take to change the situation(s) you wrote down? What would be just the first step? This is the time when fear can tighten its grip. Breathe. You don't have to do a thing. Sometimes, wrist pain or wrist injuries are simply a sign to slow down. If/when we break a bone, it can be a signal to quite literally take a break.[26]

Has your wrist pain made you modify your behavior? Be flexible with yourself.

Has your wrist pain given you the opportunity to wave hello to some help from your angels? (friends, loved ones, and spirit beings) How would it feel to ask for help?

Has your wrist pain curtailed any of your activities? How does it feel to wave goodbye for a short time?

As wrist pain gets our attention, consider it one of the TAP TAP lessons. Pause to reflect on the purpose of your pain, knowing there is a reason. Your fill-in-the-blank sentences give you a clue. While you are experiencing this distraction, understand the pause is also giving you an opportunity to reconsider if all is as you would like it to be. Your wrist pain says, *Pardon the interruption, but here's the gift of a change in your routine.* Is it time for a shift?

And so it is. And so it will be.

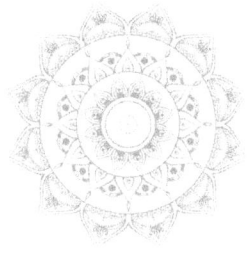

CHAPTER 8

THE GLUTES

Anger is an acid that can do more harm to the vessel in which it is stored than to anything on which it is poured.

~ Mark Twain

A Hot Pain In the A$$ - Madison

It had been about 10 minutes since our session ended, and Madison hadn't emerged from the treatment room. It was close to 9 pm so it makes sense that she may have fallen asleep on the massage table. I listened at the door. I could hear her breathing deeply.

Standing outside the door, I knocked loudly three times. I heard some movement, and then a quiet, "Yep, I'm awake." That was a bit odd. Sure, it's late in the day, but she was out.

Before the session began, Madison explained that her right glute was on fire. She had experienced this kind of pain before but could usually work through it. But not this time. She said it felt like a hot poker stabbing her in the butt. She couldn't ignore it. She had already been to an appointment with the doctor. After a 5-minute visit, which consisted of a series of verbal questions and no physical exam, he prescribed a muscle relaxer. She didn't like taking medicine but acquiesced, for now, because nothing else had worked.

Madison was a former college athlete. She played basketball and graduated with a degree in International Business. At college, she met her husband.

After college, they moved away because Ross was offered a good job with a big financial firm. Once settled in, Madison was going to explore joining the executive team of a non-profit. But that plan was put on hold as they started a family. They were blessed with a boy and a girl.

After a few years, Ross wanted to be closer to his family back home. This had been the topic of many long, tense conversations. Madison had a life. She loved being a mom and found her rhythm at the kids' school doing fundraising for their sports teams. When she talked about the events she ran, she glowed. She had been very successful, raising record amounts of money.

Madison finally gave in. Ross received a good job offer, and before the kids started high school, they moved home. The transition was difficult. The truth was, she felt like she didn't really get a vote. His job paid the bills and allowed her to be a stay-at-home mom.

During her massage session, her phone kept buzzing. She received about 20 text messages. Eventually, she asked me to hand her the phone. She sent a quick text and then turned off the phone. As she tossed it back onto a chair, she said, "What a pain in the ass." She had mentioned she'd been dealing with some extra stress lately but didn't go into details.

A light bulb went off for me. I wondered who her "pain in the ass" was. Because, quite literally, she was dealing with pain in her butt. Maybe that would be a topic for another day. My job was to address the physical imbalances in her lower back, gluteal muscles, and hamstrings. That day, she wanted (and needed) to relax.

The Lesson

The glutes represent unexpressed anger. Was Madison repressing some anger? She was.

The right side represents our masculine energy. Did she have some unexpressed anger directed toward a male? She did. She was angry at Ross.

The annoyance started when they first moved away. She felt frustrated that her husband prioritized his career over hers. She wanted to work. Ross wanted to start a family. So they did.

She adjusted and experienced success building friendships. She wanted to put down roots. Ross wanted to move. So they did.

Madison felt anger and resentment, but they had two kids to raise. She told herself that her dreams and ambitions could wait until they had an empty nest. But the emotional and social stresses were showing up in her body as glute pain. Her body was telling a different story.

After I knocked on the door just a few minutes later, Madison walked down the hallway with a confident stride. At the front desk, I offered her a bottle of water. We chatted for a few minutes. I wanted to make sure she was coherent enough to drive. (After a massage, clients can sometimes feel like they are in a haze. The relaxation response during a massage may slow down fine motor skills.) Her pupils were tiny, but she spoke clearly and was aware of her surroundings.

She handed me her credit card for payment and said she was feeling much better. She'd sleep well that night but returned with the same glute pain the following week.

Over the next few sessions, I learned that the extra stress she was talking about was that her marriage was ending. That was a surprise. Mediation was already scheduled for the end of the month. The 21-year marriage was going to end. And Madison was pissed.

Ross was trying to get full custody of the kids, citing she was misusing her pain medication. She expressed her rage. Hell hath no fury like Madison fighting for her kids. Ross had by coincidence, reconnected with an old flame. She didn't even care about the other woman. Well, she did, but that was secondary. He was trying to ruin her reputation.

She got her own lawyer. She expressed her anger. She stood up for herself. He moved out. And here's some magic: she continued to speak highly of Ross to the kids. She worked her way through her rage and took the high road.

Madison arrived for a massage late in the afternoon on the Friday of her mediation. Once in the privacy of the massage treatment room, I asked her, "How are you?"

She started to cry. She was so relieved. She got everything she asked for. She got alimony. She got child support. And she got dual custody. This was the outcome she hoped for. It seemed like a miracle. It was the vision she held in the midst of massive emotional turmoil.

Madison said she was so glad she had scheduled a massage. Her nerves were frazzled, but overall, she was doing much better.

When I asked about the right-side glute pain, she said it hadn't bothered her. I smiled. Now that the emotional stress had been relieved, her body could recalibrate. She could emotionally rebalance and heal.

The Lesson: Unexpressed Anger

Buddha (563-483 BC), the founder of Buddhism, said, "You will not be punished for your anger. You will be punished by your anger."[27]

Fast forward to 1982, when author Louise Hay released her book *Heal Your Body*. She brings to light the direct connection between the mind and body in this insightful work. She explains to future generations that there is no need to keep adding to this list even with the discovery of new previously unknown diseases. Her point is simple and echoes what has been said for hundreds of years, "I've learned that there are really two mental patterns that contribute to dis-ease: fear and anger."[28]

When we look beyond the obvious physical reasons for pain, we have the opportunity to ask, "Are there any hidden, currently undetected root causes contributing to this glute (butt) pain?' Consider *your own biography*. What's been going on? What happens to your body when you don't express your fear and anger? You may clench your teeth. Simultaneously, you may also clench your buttocks and tighten your vagina/scrotum. The emotional connection is very real.

Tension or pain in the glutes can represent unexpressed anger. Old or new, unexpressed anger can get stuck in the butt. Certainly, this isn't a one-size-fits-all explanation. Clenching the glutes is an internal response to stress. Much like unconsciously clenching the teeth, the muscular contraction in the lower back happens without thinking.

Ready to explore more of the internal landscape as it relates to glute pain? Let's start with common phrases.

He is such a pain in the butt!
I'm working my butt off on this project.
She is always butting into the conversation.

Do any of these idioms resonate with you?

Let's follow the trail of physical clues. Is the pain on the left or right side? We explore our masculine and feminine nature to understand the deeper meanings of glute pain. The right brain controls the left side of the body. The right brain functions with more intuitive feelings. The right brain tends to be thinking in a creative, holistic way. Pain on the left side of the body speaks of feminine nature. If your pain is on the left, you can ask, "Do I have unexpressed anger about a female or a traditionally feminine role? Is there a feminine energy in your life that is a pain in the butt?"

The left brain is the rational, analytical, and mathematical part of the brain. The left brain houses the more masculine traits, but it also controls the right side of the body. If your pain is on the right, you can ask, "Do I have unexpressed anger about a male? Am I angry about a traditionally male role?" Is there a masculine energy in your life that is a pain in the butt?

Let's also look at this from another angle. When you joke with words like "Oh, he's such a pain in the butt," who are you talking about? Family? Co-worker? Boss? Consider the person who sparks the irritation and butt clenching. Does the thought of this person make you growl? Sigh? Roll your eyes? Good! Now, we are getting somewhere.

Forgiveness

What's the next step, then? Whatever came to mind, it's time to forgive. Forgive and stop retelling the story. Let it go. Not ready to forgive? That's okay. However, forgiveness is not for *them*. Forgiveness is for *you*.

New Thought pastor Reverend Mark Lord recommends saying this out loud, "May forgiveness set me and everyone free.

May forgiveness set me and everyone free. May forgiveness set me and everyone free."[29] Yes, low back pain in the glutes can be scary. It's scary that we seem to have no control over it. I assure you, your intuition and your heart know what to do.

Traditional Approaches to Lower Back Pain

Lower back pain can be related to the glutes. Let's cover a few non-pharmacological approaches to treat your lower back pain. You have options beyond muscle relaxers and anti-inflammatory medicine. Some doctors recommend physical therapy, massage therapy, and even yoga to help. Ladies, consider looking for a physical therapist who specializes in pelvic floor dysfunction. Ask your Physical Therapist about the connection between jaw pain and low back pain. An underlying cause of hip/glute pain is found in the connection between the jaw and the pelvis. Elyse Shafarman, in her 2014 article for the Bodyproject.com, cited a 2009 study conducted in Germany. The study discovered that by treating jaw pain, it significantly increased the range of motion in the hips. [30] You can also consider treatment from an Osteopath (D.O.) who understands this relationship. D.O.'s regularly treat the jaw to address hip/glute pain.

In yoga, experienced instructors are taught to offer information during hip-opening poses. Hip-opening poses are sometimes part of a deeper tension pattern related to anger. Students may be surprised to feel aggravated and annoyed while holding hip-opening poses. Your yoga instructor will gently offer the point of view that as you sit with your aggravation, you are learning how to be tolerant of it in the real world. You are developing your patience. The annoyed feelings sometimes persist even after releasing the pose. Knowledgeable instructors will create a safe space for unexpressed anger and appropriate information to help process it.

Stabbed In the Back - Len

Len came to me to relieve his acute mid-shoulder back pain. He had been self-treating at home using the tennis-ball-in-a-sock method. He would place a tennis ball into a sock and throw it over his shoulder, then sandwich the ball between his back and the wall and press with some considerable effort to calm the muscle.

Do you know that spot? The one you can't quite reach that feels like a little dagger in your back. This trigger point is a classic. Many people experience pain in this area.

For Len, the pain in his back was a message from his body. He was a busy real estate agent. Len went to the gym several times a week and most days was a healthy eater. He ran his team efficiently; everyone understood their role.

While driving to work one afternoon, Len saw some real estate signs dotting his route. They looked like his signs, but with a phone number he didn't recognize. So, he called the number.

Recently, he hit a setback when one of his agents left the team to go out on their own. She was a top producer, and Len was sorry to lose her. In front of the team, Len wished her well and blessed her decision. Privately, he was pissed. He had taught her everything he knew. He paid for special training because her success was his success. As she became more successful, she relied on the entire team's help juggling all the additional responsibilities like paperwork, maintaining the database, following up on leads, and even hosting open houses. It was his marketing that gave her the leads. Normally, Len is a good forecaster; he can see what's coming. But he was completely shocked when she announced her plans to leave his brokerage.

How in the world was she going to maintain that pace by herself? But she was prepared; she was hiring her own team.

She gave her notice just as the busy season was about to start. She'd gotten a new cell phone number and was soliciting clients. The rest of the team had no idea she was planning to become a competitor. They were also surprised by her decision. Len was stunned by the premeditated planning. As a business owner, he knew these things happened but felt betrayed.

This classic tale leads to the classic trigger point. Len felt stabbed in the back. His body was telling the truth even if outwardly he was taking the high road, wishing his former team member well.

⌁ Exercise: Express Anger ⌁

Version One

As you acknowledge the origins of your glute pain, I give you permission to be right back in the situation or even in their presence. Normally, I would ask that we don't retell this kind of story that puts another person in a negative light, but today, it's okay. It's necessary to name it to reframe it. Once we finish this exercise, I invite you not to retell the story. Because retelling the story is, to your emotional self, the same as reliving the story. So the good news is this will probably be one of the last times you'll revisit that scene.

1. Think back to the time and place when you held back your anger. What did you want to say? What would you say now? Here's your opportunity.

2. Say it now. Out loud. It may feel weird or awkward, but growth doesn't happen in the comfort zone. Maybe you don't have a private space to speak out loud. Grab your journal and write it out. If it's safe and possible, don't wait. This is good stuff! Speaking out loud to express your anger is very healthy.

Version Two

Let's role-play it. Out loud.

1. Imagine the person sitting in a chair. You are somewhere safe.
2. Now, let 'em have it.

What does unexpressed anger look like? It could be loud, but it could be soft. Maybe this is new to you, so let it out of your mind. Good for you. You can speak the words. Stomp your feet. Throw your hands in the air. Make a loud noise. Sigh really loud, AAAAAHHHHH. This may seem unusual, but it's a potent way to release unexpressed anger.

Version Three

For my readers who enjoy physical expression, here's an idea. You can hit something. No, not someone. *Something.*

Hit a heavy bag at your gym. Hit a pillow sitting on the chair. Throw a punch in the air. Of course, be careful of your hands. We are being mindful of the way we express ourselves. Staying safe, but *getting it out of your system.*

You are releasing punch by punch, the energy that has been pent up inside you for a long time, in theory, long enough to give you pain in your glutes. By intentionally hitting a heavy bag, we can intentionally release the stuck and, therefore unexpressed emotions. We punch out the pain in the butt! This process can reveal the story your pain is trying to tell you. The body's internal mechanisms may seem like a mystery, but the mystery can be revealed when we explore and listen to our emotions, our beautiful internal compass.

Version Four

Pause for a moment. Maybe you are an in control person. Acting out dramatically feels uncomfortable or a little too raw for you. Fair enough.

1. Ask yourself a simple question: "What am I learning from this pain in my butt?" Then, sit still. No distractions. No TV. No book or magazine. No phone. Sit still.

2. Let your eyes close and listen to your breath. With your windows to the world (eyes) shut, ask again, "What am I learning from this pain in the butt?" Does someone's face come to mind? Do you hear your inner voice saying, *slow down*? Do you see color?

These are part of your message, my friend. You may not fully understand yet, but your answers are coming.

One of my heroes, Nelson Mandela, said,

Courage is not the absence of fear, but the triumph over it.
The brave man is not he who does not feel afraid,
but he who conquers that fear.

I wish you the courage to act, forgive, and let it go. To do whatever it is that is yours to do.

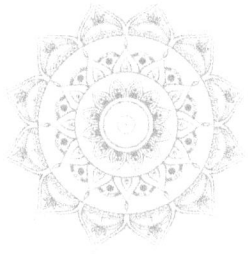

CHAPTER 9

THE KNEES

*I love you when you bow in your mosque, kneel in
your temple, pray in your church. For you and I are sons
of one religion, and it is the spirit.*

~ Khalil Gibran (1883-1931)
author of The Prophet

Bowing Down - Kevin

Kevin has had knee pain off and on for many of his 25 years. He was a rock star baseball catcher in high school and college. Minor League Baseball looked certain. Major leagues looked possible. Kevin eventually became a very talented, driven personal trainer. This is where our paths crossed. Kevin is my trainer for the day. After what seemed like endless push-ups (it was only 15), Kevin asked, "So you're writing a book about the meaning of pain in different parts of the body?" I'm panting and can't form a complete sentence, so I nod. He's curious, "What do knees mean?" After I catch my breath, I explain.

Knees are used to kneel. Sometimes, that leads to kneeling down and bowing, let's say bending, against our wills. Traditionally, we kneel when we pray or to show respect. For example, even today, when famous people meet the King of England, they bend their knees to bow or curtsy. Little did I know that Kevin had his own version of a Monarch in his castle. He went on to explain he'd had quite a bit of knee pain over the years due to the challenging physical demands of baseball. His pain would come and go. Over the last year, his knees had started to bother him again regularly. I assured him that his knee pain was most likely rooted in the hours he spent crouched behind home plate.

He looked pensive, then admitted, "Normally, I would have agreed with you. Now that I'm thinking about it, I've had almost no knee pain in the last six months." He became lost in thought and said, "It was about six months ago that my girlfriend and I broke up. She always needed to be in control. When we would go out, she would get really jealous if I talked to anyone else. Seems like too big of a coincidence to ignore, doesn't it?"

I smiled and nodded. Indeed. Maybe the pain was caused by years of being in the squatting position as a catcher, or his knees were trying to get his attention to say, *stop being a pushover*. It was likely a combination of both. But he was now living pain-free.

The Lesson: Bending of the Will

Knees are about bending. Knee pain can indicate bending more than we like or want to. Knee pain can represent resentment over bending against our will. Physically, the knees are the joining point between our upper and lower legs, which speaks to elevating our current situation. The knee joint allows the rising up from the lower leg to the upper leg from one level to the next. Knee pain can represent the fear of going from a lower position to a higher position. Knee pain could indicate a reluctance to change.

Healthy knees are flexible. They bend smoothly. Healthy knees have a full range of motion. As we know this about our knees, we can know this for our lives. If we get curious about these movements in our lives, we can ask ourselves, *Where could I be more flexible? Where could I smooth things over? Where do I need to have a fuller range of motion or widen my circle of acceptance?*

Louise Hay writes about the knees representing our stubborn ego and pride.[31] Our inability or unwillingness to bend. Emily A. Francis, in her book *The Body Heals Itself*, associates knees with being the messenger of how you are experiencing change. According to Francis, being rigid or being at a standstill could be the source of some of your knee pain.[32]

In my research and experience, I have found some more specific meanings for knee pain. What do knees do? Knees bend. Why do knees bend? We bend to kneel and to show respect. Down on two knees, we kneel to pray. We kneel to surrender. Kneeling is a symbolic representation of bending our wills. Why do we bend our wills? At times, we bend or surrender to show deference, respect, or compromise.

Knee Treatment Options

Acupuncture and other treatments used by TCM have been proven effective at increasing the range of motion and decreasing swelling, as well as treating Osteoarthritis. By treating the "kidney deficiency, blood stagnation and the retention of damp cold in the knees," TCM can help avoid needing a total knee replacement.[33] Who do you know that gets acupuncture? Ask them for a referral.

By the way, knee surgery is rarely a silver bullet. About *half* of my clients who had their knees replaced experienced serious pain and needed long-term physical therapy. A 2017 British Medical Journal article, *Impact of Total Knee Replacement Practice: Cost-Effectiveness Analysis of Date from the Osteoarthritis Initiative,* offers some data. The study documents the experience of 4,498 patients. Approximately 1/3 saw "minimal effects on quality of life" after their knee replacement.[34] *Minimal effects* on improving the quality of life? That is, in my opinion, no bueno. Only 33% found they benefited from the surgery. That sounds like a good reason to avoid surgery or to at least exhaust all other alternatives.

As of 2023, progress is being made to help improve outcomes. In some hospitals, robotics are used to assist during the surgery. Studies are finding the robot-assisted surgeries are leading to better alignment, shorter recovery times, and better results. That is good news!

Knee pain responds exceptionally well to specific massage therapy techniques and specialized physical therapy. When knee pain becomes chronic and recurs frequently, try calling on a highly qualified massage therapist and/or physical therapist. Have them work the soft tissue around the knee. Ultimately, you may need to have the joint replaced, but massage and PT can relieve the current symptoms and help balance the joint prior to surgery.

⌒ The Exercise: Bowing Down or Standing Up ⌒

To help you determine if there could be a biopsychosocial connection to why *your* knee hurts, ask yourself some simple questions.

Where am I bending my will?

Who is the person that I would rather not bend to, but I don't want to make a fuss?

What duty am I being asked to fulfill? Is it truly my duty?

Who am I bowing down to? Is there a king or queen in my life? Where am I bowing down too often?

If I could have my own way with something, what would it be?

Where could I be more flexible? Where might I benefit from showing more respect?

What is making me weak in the knees?

Where do I feel like I can't stand up for myself?

1. Write down any emotions you are feeling. Pay attention to your discomfort. This is a good sign that it's true for you. Part of healing from physical pain is addressing the biopsychosocial reasons for your pain. Understanding the mental, emotional, and/or social root causes is part of excavating the source of chronic pain. True recovery is possible when we are open to the message(s) our pain has to tell us.

2. Ask yourself, *What am I to learn from this pain*? Be still. Ask again, *What is there for me to learn from this pain?*

3. Breathe. Listen to the still, small voice inside of you. It's been quiet for some time. Would you be willing to make some space to listen?

Knee pain often is a combination of several challenges. My experience demonstrates there is almost always an underlying biopsychosocial involvement with knee pain. Perhaps ask one more question. Is there anyone I need to forgive? Almost always, there's someone. Trust me; I *still* cringe at the forgiveness question. When I think I've done all the forgiving I have to do, there is always someone else. Sometimes, I just have to forgive myself. Forgiveness is where all healing begins.

Sending love and light. Hope your knees feel better.

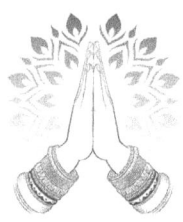

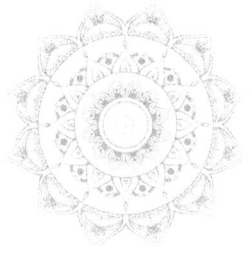

CHAPTER 10

THE ANKLES

*The art of life lies in a constant readjustment
to our surroundings.*

~ Kakuzo Okakura,
Japanese Scholar

Hard-headed - Mary

My friend's mom, Mary, started experiencing ankle pain. She went to her local doctor, who ordered an X-ray. Nothing wrong. A friend referred her for a massage. During our session, I learned that Mary is a proud, hard-working woman. She shared that about three months prior, she had discovered that her husband had taken on yet another girlfriend. For Mary, that was the last one she would bear. She was furious and embarrassed. Mary was feeling twenty-plus years of frustration all at once. She had recently filed for divorce. When it came time to figure out the finances of the divorce, Mary said she wanted to spit in his face. That is not the ideal frame of mind for negotiations.

During the divorce mediation, she told her soon-to-be ex-husband she wanted nothing from him. Her mind wandered and she imagined him taking credit for supporting her. This made her blood boil. She didn't want any handouts. While I understand her self-reliant spirit, her stubborn pride blinded her judgment. Mary wanted him out of her life for good. Yet her anger was sabotaging her future. Pride can feel overwhelming and create complete inflexibility. The ancient philosopher, Khalil Gibran offers this point of view, "Generosity is giving more than you can; Pride is taking less than you need."

Because of her inflexibility, Mary struggled financially for almost a decade to *get back on her feet*. Could being more flexible have made her life a little easier? I think so. That struggle was more difficult than it had to be because of her inflexibility. Strong emotions are a big red flag that you aren't in the best frame of mind to make decisions. Step back and breathe. We did get Mary's ankle pain under control. And now, she is more willing to be flexible with bumpy circumstances. When she looks back at that situation, she has compassion for herself. She felt betrayed. She knows in the face of such strong emotions today, she would make different decisions.

The Lesson: Adjust to Changing Terrain

Katherine Woodward Thomas introduced the United States to the concept of Conscious Uncoupling in 2011. If you have strong emotions around the transition of your relationship, you can take your power back. According to Thomas, your gift to yourself will be "happy even after."[35]

Chronic ankle pain often has a story to tell beyond the ligaments and tendons. Hay refers to ankles as representing inflexibility and guilt. In my experience, ankles represent someone who has been digging their heels in over a certain situation. Ankles help us balance. The ankle is a multi-directional joint where we adjust to the terrain of life. Imagine walking or jogging on a trail in the woods. Your ankles help to accommodate the rocks and swollen tree roots poking out of the ground. Watch carefully, or you might trip. You may slow your pace a little when these obstacles show up to allow your ankles time to adjust. Your ankles allow you to roll with the ups and downs of the path.

What unexpected stumbling blocks have you encountered lately? Have you tripped? Not literally, but figuratively. I have literally tripped more than once while happily jogging. One such time was while working with some of the world's fastest, most talented Track and Field athletes at the World Athletic Championships in Japan. I was inspired by being surrounded by so much talent! So off I went for a jog around Osaka Castle. I was enjoying the scenery, feeling grateful when slam! My toe hit a root, and I was stopped in my tracks, skidding on the ground on my hands and knees. Was it the tree's fault I fell? No. The tree didn't trip me on purpose. Oh, for sure, I had all the normal feelings. *Am I okay? Did anyone see that?* I felt ridiculous and clumsy. I mostly laughed at myself because none of the Japanese people passing me even made eye contact. This was proper behavior for Japanese culture – don't acknowledge the fall. Ignore it and just keep walking. There are no major concerns, just a bit of broken skin on the heels of my hands and knees. I got up, dusted off, slowed down, and started walking.

The lessons that unfolded over the next ten days were going to be quite challenging, and I would need to be very flexible. Solid advice. I was working at the World Championships of Track & Field in Osaka Japan. I was in a foreign country, in an area that didn't speak much English. My Japanese was limited to simple words of courtesy. Everything was unfamiliar. I felt out of place and insecure. That trip taught me to be flexible, whether I wanted to be or not. I believe things happen for a reason. In hindsight, I could appreciate the message of my trip over that tree root: Slow down, be flexible, and adjust.

Do both of your ankles have pain? Is there a situation in your life where you just refuse to discuss options? Have you dug in your heels and are completely inflexible?

Having both ankles in pain is unusual, so remember to rule out any significant physical conditions. Schedule a visit to a qualified Physical Therapist, Orthopedic doctor, or Sports Chiropractor.

⌁ The Exercise: Know Thyself ⌁

Exercise One

If you have chronic pain in your ankles, start by examining the pain.

1. Notice when the pain started. Did the pain start after a long walk, after a race, after a fall, after an accident, or did the dog jerk you on the leash? Did you try a new activity (ski, snowboard, surf, skateboard)? Answering yes could indicate a purely physical issue. If not, continue asking questions.

2. *When* do you have ankle pain? Morning? All day? At night? After standing all day? Again, this could indicate a purely physical condition. If there is no specific time of day for the pain, let's investigate a little more.

3. Is the pain sharp or dull when it happens? Pretty sharp? Yes? Keep reading.

4. Is the pain on the left or right side?

   As we know, the left side indicates a feminine issue. Is there a situation in your life involving a female where you could be more flexible? What would it look like if you expanded your thinking to be just 1% more flexible? What if you were 5% more flexible? Respect your own boundaries; be aware of strong emotions.

   As we have learned, the right side indicates a masculine issue. Is there a situation in your life where you are being inflexible that involves a male? What would it look like if you were just 1% more flexible? What if you were 5% more flexible.

5. Breathe. Let your eyes close. Listen.

At this point, you might know where you are being inflexible. To take a baby step forward, ask yourself, *How could I act with love in this situation?* How could you show up as love, with love, from a place of love. Yes, this is work, but you will get there. Or you won't, right now. It's all good. One reminder: Showing up with love is not for someone else. Showing up with love is for *you*. As we do the personal work to understand the story pain is telling us, I am reminded of a Universal rule: My life lesson is never about anyone else outside myself. It's almost always about me.

Exercise Two

Affirmations for the ankle.

1. Say out loud

   a. I am flexible.
   b. I am willing to change and see every situation for how it serves me.
   c. Life happens *for* me.
   d. I accept all the good that is coming to me.
   e. I deserve joy and happiness in my life.

Is ankle pain physical or is it mental? It's usually a combination of the two. Yes, you may have had ten sprained ankles while playing lacrosse in college as one client explained. However, even with stretched tendons, chronic ankle pain often tells us more. There is a story being revealed by the persistent pain getting your attention. You now have much of the information you need to treat that physical, mental, or emotional ankle pain. Good for you!

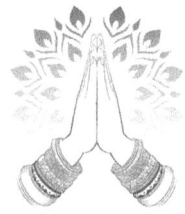

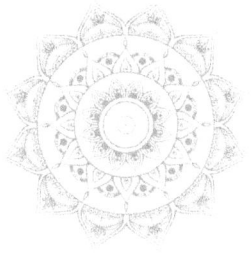

CHAPTER 11

THE FEET

*Real change, enduring change, happens
one step at a time.*

~ Ruth Bader Ginsburg

Earth Signs - Jeremiah

Jeremiah paused as he climbed down the pool ladder. His girlfriend Jada saw him pause and was curious, "Is the water cold?" He shakes his head. The steps of the ladder were gritty and grooved, and it felt like little knives stabbing into his feet. Maybe if he stood very still, it wouldn't hurt. Jeremiah was almost never barefoot. Just the idea of walking without shoes on the sidewalk sent shivers down his spine. Pool ladders were his kryptonite. He thought wearing pool shoes was silly, but after this experience, he might have to set aside his fashion sense and get a pair.

As a young kid, Jeremiah had spent hours at the gym boxing. A tough and intelligent kid from the mean streets of suburbia, he found the gym to be a second home. A long-time swimmer, he had always used the locker room showers after his workout. He thought other guys wearing sandals in the shower looked weird. Why bother? Gyms can be a breeding ground for fungi, viruses and bacteria. These can cause warts, ringworm, the spread of flu and staph infections.

Unfortunately, it wasn't long until plantar warts covered the bottoms of his feet. A family friend, a retired podiatrist, was asked to take care of the issue. It was the 1980s – friends helping friends. So he sat in a recliner in his dad's living room as the doctor rolled out his tools, including a scalpel, and began to dig and cut. The job must have taken most of the afternoon because when he was done, the sun was setting, and he could smell his mom cooking dinner. No more warts, but Jeremiah's feet were on fire. His feet had been hyper-sensitive ever since.

His mind wandered as he stood very still on the second step of the pool ladder. This vacation gave him time to consider his life in general. He had risen as high as the company he worked for would allow in his current position. The money was good, and he was good at it. But he was bored. Jeremiah had recently decided to look around to explore other options. He had stretched and applied for a position with a firm where he hoped to get an offer, but he wasn't sure if he should take the leap. He'd be the new guy. He'd have to prove himself all over again. What if it didn't work out? He knew eventually, it would be time to move on, but he was scared of making a mistake. Maybe he should stay in the secure, safe, boring, well-paying job now.

When he returned home from the pool, Jeremiah got the offer from the new firm. It was an entry-level position, but there was a lot of upward mobility. He took the leap. The first year was a blur, getting used to brand-new technology and the personalities of his new colleagues. But the challenge was exciting and, while exhausting, fun.

Foot pain represents being afraid to take the next step in life. Jeremiah's courage paid off with an offer from a nationally known company. He increased his take-home pay by 30% - even after taxes. He finally took his next steps, said yes to the offer, and found some relief mentally and physically by having the guts to move forward.

His new position gave him better insurance, so he also explored new strategies that addressed the physical, mental, and emotional layers of his pain. He started to see a therapist, and the therapist suggested Jeremiah visit one new place, each month that he'd never been before.

This was a stretch. Jeremiah preferred to stick with what he knew. He took baby steps. He and Jada tried a new restaurant. He found out he liked Thai food. Trying something new each month made Jeremiah more comfortable saying yes to other new opportunities.

When a 2-year assignment within the company became available in California, he shocked his friends and family by accepting. He had always wanted to explore the west coast. The transition was exciting, and Jeremiah even had to start pacing himself. Now, he enjoys the awesome weather year-round. His foot pain has disappeared. He even started hiking on the weekends with a local group in Orange County. Today, he and his longtime girlfriend Jada, own two homes, one on the west coast and the other on the east coast. Just the other day, he found himself window-shopping for rings. Maybe it's time to make another bold leap?

Ticklish Feet

Maybe your feet are not in pain, but they feel ticklish. Ticklish feet can be a sign of not feeling connected to the place you are in. For example, do you feel connected to your home? At your workplace? Where do you feel like a fish out of water? If you answer everywhere, that feeling of disconnection can be represented by having ticklish feet.

One easy way to feel more connected to where you are is to go barefoot. Well, maybe not at work. But when do you go barefoot? Getting in and out of the shower? Getting up in the morning? Some of my clients tell me it's too painful to go barefoot. I understand. We may have to work a little harder to find pleasing ways for our feet to connect with the ground. How about on a furry rug? Maybe in the soft sand with waves licking at your toes? Even just imagining this connection to the Earth (with your shoes on) can create a feeling of being grounded.

The ticklish feeling in the feet can also originate from a feeling of being disconnected from your present circumstances. Do you spend a lot of time in your head? Many of us do. Is it hard to tell? Here are a few clues.

Do you lose track of time when you are online? Remedy: Set an alarm every 30 minutes to stand up, change your gaze, feel your feet, wiggle your toes, getting grounded in the present moment.

Do you find yourself spacing out while driving? Remedy: When you arrive at your destination, pause either in the vehicle or outside the car. Take two minutes to breathe. Plant your feet on the ground and take in your surroundings. Are there birds singing? Are there clouds in the sky?

These little habits can make you more productive and create a feeling of being more tuned in to where you're going and who you're seeing.

The Lesson: Staying Grounded

Foot pain gives us a chance to ask, "What are my next steps? Or "Is it time to walk away?" Maybe you have felt like you are taking one step forward and two steps back. If you are experiencing foot pain with a biopsychosocial connection, when asking these questions, your gut reaction often comes quickly. To make a change may take a little longer. Lao Tzu says, "The journey of a thousand miles starts with one step." [36] What is one small step you could take today related to moving forward?

Are you familiar with the term *getting grounded*? This is different from being grounded as punishment, and it's different from avoiding an electrical shock. This term refers to feeling a connection to the Earth. Feeling your feet on the ground. Being present, here and now.

The challenge to staying grounded is that, as mentioned earlier, most of us spend a lot of time in our heads. It's easy to feel disconnected from the here and now. How many times have you asked yourself, *What day is it?* I find myself saying, *It's still Monday?* Sometimes, the best remedy to feeling scattered is to take a short walk in nature. Sometimes, you don't have the option to stop everything you are doing and take a walk. Remedy: You could put a walk on the schedule. Research has proven that uninterrupted time to think is highly valuable. AOL's CEO Tim Armstrong asks that his executives spend four hours a week just thinking.[37] CEO of LinkedIn, Jeff Weiner, schedules two hours of uninterrupted time every day to think.[38]

So where is the balance? Having time to think is beneficial. One of the reasons we have great ideas in the bathroom or the shower is because alone, uninterrupted we can think. And our feet are firmly connected to the ground. The *challenge* comes when we spend time in our heads obsessing and worrying about the past or the future. Staying grounded involves staying in the present moment. Physically pressing your feet into the ground, you can tune into your feet simply by bringing your attention there. Stretching your toes, curling your toes, wiggling your toes. Feeling the bottoms of your feet touching your shoes or the ground. If you are in stocking feet, you can touch your toes. Put your thumb on your arch and give that area a light pinch. With your hand on your foot, you can notice how your feet feel.

When I'm not grounded, I've been known to forget where I put my keys, drive away with coffee on top of the car or look for the cell phone that is in my hand at my ear.

Whether you have ticklish feet or feel foot pain, I encourage you, at different times of the day, to get grounded. Get back in your body and out of your head by tuning into your feet.

⌁ The Exercise: Feel Your Feet ⌁

How do you get grounded? Focusing on the breath is one of my favorite techniques.

1. In a comfortable position, plant your feet on the ground and wiggle your toes. Tune in for a moment to your body. Take a deep breath. Hold for a few seconds. You are here, present in your body. You are grounded.

2. Whether you're barefoot or in shoes, tune in and feel the bottoms of your feet. Rub your feet back and forth. Curl your toes. Stretch your toes wide. Really focus on your feet. Press into the ground below you. Take a breath.

This is one of the easiest ways to get back to the present moment. We live busy lives; *who has time* to consciously get present or feel grounded? Aside from a few special monks, no one has time to sit and meditate all day. Here's the difference. We don't *have* time. We *make* time.

We make time to ask simple questions. We make time to get grounded. We make time to be present because making time to explore the biopsychosocial connections may be the key to relieving your foot pain

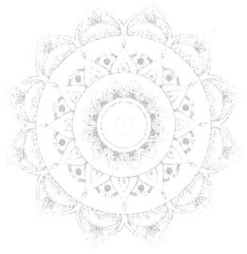

CHAPTER 12

RASH OR HIVES

Natural forces within us are the true healers of disease.

~ Hippocrates (460 BC to 370 BC)

Tough Chick - Katherine

Massage therapy sometimes sneaks in behind the rigid external walls we have built to stay safe. A nurturing, kind touch may allow a person to process the next cycle of healing. This was the case with one of my tough chick clients. I knew Katherine to be a no-nonsense woman. She was warm, yet she was always in control of her emotions. In one session, she surprised both of us when she began to cry. The tears quietly rolled down her temples. Her body and mind felt safe to release something. Specifically what, neither of us knew.

The next morning, Katherine called to offer me some feedback, "Hey, I'm very happy with my massage, but my chest broke out in little red bumps after our session. What do you think of that?" She assured me she wasn't alarmed, just curious.

I shared with her that rashes represent the exit of lots of little hidden fears. She confirmed that metaphorical meaning made sense to her. Over the summer, she experienced quite a bit of loss. Recently, she had learned another loss may be on the horizon. A good friend of hers, young like her, just shared shocking news. After over a year of good health, a friend she admired and looked up to had just been diagnosed again with cancer. This news reinforced Katherine's fears about her sense of safety and peace in the world. It reinforced her unspoken fear that bad things happen to good people. This didn't make sense. She believed in karma and that good things happen to good people. She didn't share everything that she was processing with me, but the rash revealed that there was a lot going on.

Interestingly, the rash she developed hovered only above her heart area. No other parts of her chest or body broke out into a rash. Once Katherine and I spoke about the possible meaning and origin of the rash, it calmed down almost immediately. The hot bumps were gone the next day. Her condition was a flash message, a quick tap for Katherine to acknowledge and release some of her hidden fears.

The Lesson: Little Worries

The Father of Medicine, Hippocrates, understood we are wired to be well. The sympathetic nervous system activates the fight or flight system, which regulates our body's reaction to stress. Depending on how often and for how long you have been handling confrontation determines some of the body's external responses. Hives and rashes are a classic reaction to stress. Ask yourself, "Did the rash (or hives) appear at a specific time?" Sure, it could be a reaction to some food you ate. It also could be a sign of deeper processing going on. Itchy, hot bumps may mean your body is trying to get your attention.

A rash can be caused by a host of different physical reasons. Yet, before we sound the alarm and diagnose ourselves with an unlikely physical condition, let's consider what research tells us about the biopsychosocial reasons for a rash. Current research has documented a strong connection between unusually high levels of mental stress and the onset of a physical rash.

The biopsychosocial method isn't named specifically by the Cleveland Clinic's publication *Health Essentials*, but, in essence, the author reports that stress hives are a real medical condition.[39] Mental stress causes physical symptoms. For some, a rash represents the mental equivalent of a temper tantrum. Questions racing through your brain like "What is going on here? How can she be sick again?" Imagine foot stomping as your inner child declares, "I don't want to accept this!" And, truth be told, Katherine was also worried that since her healthy spiritual friend had gotten sick again, could she get sick? Katherine was healthy and spiritual. Was she vulnerable?

Some researchers believe itchy bumps represent making mountains out of molehills, which is another manifestation of fear. Are you projecting in to the future and worried about an outcome you can't control? All breakouts offer us the opportunity to learn some important life lessons about choosing to stay present. Likewise, when we consider the future, imagine positive outcomes to combat fear.

A Caution

I want to caution you to approach this subject gently. If you, your child, partner, or best friend has a breakout, rash, or skin disruption of any kind, be compassionate. Our skin is how we show up in the world. It can feel very vulnerable when our skin isn't glowing and smooth. Some skin conditions are inherited. Even with the best medical care, the condition persists. If you have classmates, friends, or family members with psoriasis, eczema, or acne, be kind. See beyond the blemishes. Acceptance without judgment demonstrates love.

More Than Skin Deep

We are learning more and more from Medical Intuitives like Laura Bruno. I enjoyed her story about her experience of the underlying causes of rashes.[40] Let me summarize this fascinating account. Ms. Bruno dealt with a crazy, odd rash on her right thigh for a couple of months. She noticed it followed exactly the energy channel of the bladder meridian. Meridians are energy pathways used in Acupuncture and Chinese Medicine. The rash was creeping down this meridian and down her leg, so Laura decided to see a dermatologist.

The dermatologist was alarmed and immediately biopsied the area. The doctor confirmed it was a rash normally only seen on children around the age of three. This just got interesting because one of Laura's favorite people in the world, her paternal grandfather, died when she was three. She vividly remembers the day he died because so many people were hurting that she didn't express her grief in case it made everyone else upset. She still remembers drawing with him as a child.

That day she stuffed her grief and shock down far inside. Someone she loved could just disappear? In her writing on the subject, she explains that the grief "left a mark on her inner terrain" and over the years, she's worked to release this grief.

The diagnosis (lichen striatus) was not contagious, infectious or in any way dangerous. Laura realized the connection between the bladder meridian and the water element, which connects to old sadness. In reality, Laura sees this more as a "celebration in that my soul feels ready to release those traumas in a final way."

Her dermatologist still urged her to use a steroid cream, but she opted not to since that would only repress the symptoms. She explained, "If this is an old drama coming to the surface after 33 years, then it feels right to let it play itself out."

I've seen this pattern so many times in clients. They attempt to soothe or cure their symptoms when they could benefit from sitting with the discomfort to decipher and recognize the cause. There is no need to suffer with poison ivy, but if a random rash occurs, pause to consider the stress you may be experiencing. Sometimes dietary shifts or creams help, but sometimes the skin simply announces the progress being made by making visible what is occurring beneath perception. Sometimes 'ugly' skin makes us infinitely more conscious of our inner beauty and vulnerability. And whenever that happens, I rejoice.

The Exercise: Name Your Worry

Do you want to find out if there is more to your story? Grab a pen and paper and set a timer for 5 minutes. Sit in a quiet place with both your feet on the floor. Let your eyes close. Think of the area of your rash/hives.

Ask yourself,

1. What are you telling me?
2. What do you want me to know about this irritation?

3. Be in the quiet. Listen to your breath. Focus on the in and out of your breathing. What images come to mind? If outside thoughts bubble up, bless and release them. Come back as often as you like to the breath. Your only work is to sit, listen to the breath, and ask the questions.

4. Once the timer goes off, write down your thoughts. What did you learn? What actions might you take? Is it time to spend less time with that irritating client? Or a difficult family member?

After you jot down some thoughts, breathe. You are learning to listen to your body! You are listening. You are paying attention. Yay you! This is a major breakthrough. It may not seem like much right now, but your willingness to participate demonstrates you are ready to receive. Your journey of healing *from the inside out* has begun. Bravo! Good work.

CHAPTER 13

FIBROMYALGIA

Begin to see yourself as a soul with a body rather than a body with a soul.

~ Wayne Dyer

Emotionally Beat Up - Mila

Mila had always been perceived as outgoing and fun. She worked hard at her job; her colleagues respected her. No one would have guessed she was being verbally and emotionally abused at home. Her husband seemed like a nice enough guy. Of course, he had his little quirks. He washed his hands all the time and used a lot of hand sanitizer. His friends would joke with him, calling him a germaphobe. Mila's husband didn't like to fly, so he didn't take any of the adventurous family vacations with her and the kids. He always said he couldn't take time off from work.

He never laid a hand on her, but in the 20+ years after raising two children, she was unsure if she had ever felt loved or appreciated. Once the kids were in college, he became more critical of her. The verbal fault-finding was ongoing. *The house wasn't clean enough. She was lazy. She was going to set the house on fire the way she cooked.* He already worked long hours at the office, but now he was staying even later.

Mila felt strange one weekend while he was away tending to his mother. Whatever it was, it came as a surprise. She was sitting in a chair, reading a book, and she realized what the strange feeling was; she was happy. She was happy he wasn't there. She found herself daydreaming he wouldn't come home. She sat with that fascinating thought for a moment. She knew she should banish the thought, but she couldn't. She tried to stop smiling at the thought of never seeing him again.

Intellectually, she realized the relationship wasn't working, but couldn't end it. They were the perfect couple: two kids, a dog, cool vacations. Over time, her body began betraying her. She wasn't lazy - she was in pain. She hurt everywhere. Her shoulders, her back, even her legs hurt. She slept 10 hours a night but still felt exhausted. She considered going to the doctor, but what doctor? The pain would be in different places on different days. Some days, it wasn't so bad. But other days, she couldn't get out of bed. She was worried she may be really sick. What if she had the big "C"? She was stuck. Stuck in a good house, with a good car, with good insurance, and in a marriage that was making her ill.

Finally, she found the courage to go to the rheumatologist and tell her about the random, crazy, debilitating symptoms. The doctor asked a series of questions and did a physical exam. She didn't have cancer. That day, Mila learned that she had a condition called fibromyalgia. (Fi-bro-my-al-ja)

Fibromyalgia causes pain all over the body and specifically in at least 11 of 18 specific tender points. Fibromyalgia is an intricate matrix of physical symptoms and emotions that create pain all over the body.

To get a small inkling of what it's like, imagine you have been on a long trip. You are really quite ready to be at home, and your flight is canceled. It's going to be hours until the next flight. Maybe you tried to sleep in the airport sitting up in a chair. Only to wake up from a couple of hours of broken sleep, trying to remember where you are and what day it is. The feeling of being bone tired has crept in overnight, and you hurt in places you didn't know you had. All you want to do is get home and sleep in your own bed. That's a good day for a patient diagnosed with fibromyalgia.

Did you experience COVID? The physical implosion of aches, pains, and fatigue? That's an average day for some people dealing with fibromyalgia. And the deep rest never seems to come. Day after day, they soldier on. Sometimes, they feel they are going through the motions, living their lives in a blur, waiting for a ray of sunshine.

For Mila, she was relieved to know her condition had a name. Yet the doctor told her the treatment varied between patients. There were some medications, but the side effects were not pleasant. Mila didn't like taking medications. One thing that seemed consistent with every patient was that massage therapy helped relieve the pain. That proved true for Mila also; massage therapy reduced the pain and calmed her frazzled nerves.

Next, she found the courage to tell her husband she wanted a divorce. He threatened to destroy her. This divorce would be a two-year battle, but it was an important part of her healing journey. True healing includes finding peace of mind. As Mila's peace of mind increased, her confidence increased. As her time away from the toxic person increased, the fibromyalgia symptoms decreased.

Fibromyalgia impacts between 6 and 12 million people, representing about 2%-4% of the US population.[41] It affects women more than men by 9:1.[42] Fibromyalgia acts like an autoimmune disease, but it isn't. Part of what makes fibromyalgia tricky is that there doesn't seem to be one singular cause. As you can imagine, that makes it difficult to treat.

The first symptom is often extreme fatigue that a person just can't shake. It often takes months before the person goes to the doctor because they think they'll eventually get over whatever 'this' is.

In the past, fibromyalgia has been labeled a 'mystery illness.' It's becoming a little less mysterious as it becomes more recognizable. Mila's doctor referred her for massage because it's one of the few treatments that consistently helps the symptoms. Research from the Cleveland Clinic confirms that massage helps control inflammation, which is an important factor in treating fibromyalgia.[43]

Good to know, but what about the cause? In my experience, fibromyalgia is a condition having its roots in stress that causes emotional exhaustion.

The Biopsychosocial Impact

Mila had a tremendous amount of mental stress. As a result, her nervous system was regularly in fight or flight. It was her definition of normal, her day-to-day experience. As science increases our awareness of the impact of mental and emotional pressure, we can begin to appreciate that external pressure is a large part of a person's internal suffering. Pain and suffering can exhibit as exhaustion.

During the divorce, Mila worried her college aged kids would be negatively influenced by her soon to be ex-husband. They had raised smart children who saw through the exaggerations and mistruths. Dad was saying Mom was on the verge of a mental breakdown. What they witnessed was that Mom was moving on with her life. Making new friends and even taking a cooking class. The kids navigated the emotional waters of their parent's divorce. The kids stayed level headed. They loved both parents, albeit in different ways. Mila learned that her kids possessed emotional intelligence. She felt proud when they negotiated spending time with both parents during the holidays. Mila was relieved, calm and appreciative. This new chapter of her life felt better than she could have imagined.

Yet that's not the whole story of fibromyalgia. You see, it's not just mental and emotional stress causing the symptoms. Sometimes the root cause is abuse.

You're Not Alone - Hanna and Cathy

Hanna and Cathy are the new two-person team arriving to help me clean my house. Hanna sees the massage table and asks if I'm a therapist. I smile and say, "Yup." Hanna told me that she is also a massage therapist. Hanna's mom was also a Licensed Massage Therapist. She had been around massage therapy for as long as she could remember. No coincidences, right? I wondered why she wasn't practicing. It seemed odd. Soon, she would reveal why she wasn't working with clients.

As the ladies went about their work, I was pecking away at the computer, writing this book. Cathy poked her head around the corner and asked, "Hey, so what's the book about?" I gave a few simple examples of pain and its underlying meanings. Cathy got right to the point, asking if all pain has a meaning. "What does fibromyalgia mean?" Pointing to Hanna, "She has fibro." Hanna's eyes got wide, and her cheeks flushed. Hanna awkwardly explained that after massage school, she couldn't predict when her fibromyalgia was going to flare up. She felt unreliable. She was trying to build a private practice, but too often, she'd have to reschedule clients due to her pain. Eventually, she stopped seeing clients.

I was quiet. You see, this condition is different for every person who has it. Different events trigger it. I shared with them that, based on my experience, fibromyalgia can be the result of some sort of abuse. Hanna bowed her head, grabbed her broom, and started sweeping. I almost didn't hear her when she whispered, "Well, that would make sense." My job at that moment was just to plant a seed of knowledge. I could feel her discomfort, so I was surprised at her willingness to confirm her case had been born of an abusive relationship. She had ended that relationship, but the memory still stung.

I imagined love flowing out of my heart to hers. To shift the focus, I looked back at Cathy, and we grabbed our calendars to schedule for next time. But I felt the seed of knowledge take root inside Hanna. Sometimes, you can never not know, once you know. The next time I saw Hanna, she stuck out her left hand and waved it up and down. She is in a healthy, devoted relationship with a man who adores her. Her symptoms flare up occasionally, but she tells me she has never felt happier and healthier.

The Lesson: A Connection Between Abuse and Fibromyalgia

Because people often don't want to talk about it, I felt I had to include my experience working with patients diagnosed with fibromyalgia. Over the 20+ years I've been practicing massage, I've learned that there is often a connection between fibromyalgia and abuse. If abuse is a part of the patient experience (disclosed or undisclosed), the three most common types are physical abuse as a child, sexual abuse as a child, and verbal abuse/mental abuse as an adult.

If you were abused as a child, that's not okay. Professional therapy is recommended. If you are experiencing symptoms of Fibro, one of the paths to healing is to acknowledge the highs and lows of your childhood. Find and talk to a great therapist.

Verbal abuse as an adult takes many forms. Venomous comments can be poorly disguised as insulting jokes. Belittling by a partner or spouse. Judging. Criticizing. Yelling. Name-calling. Threatening. Someone who is calling you crazy or continually questioning your sanity (gaslighting). They may never raise a hand, but this is abuse.

These types of behaviors by a bully reinforce the lies being told. You are not crazy. You are beautiful. You are not inherently broken. You are perfect. You are perfect just the way you are. Sometimes, a person subject to prolonged abuse can lose sight of the truth. The manipulating aggressor has maintained a type of control because there is only so much energy and so much will to fight. We choose our battles to, hopefully, win the war. Those diagnosed with fibromyalgia often report feeling tired and worn down. The weary mind can play tricks, asking, "Are the hateful messages the truth?" No, they are not. But after months and years of being subject to negative words and actions, the body could manifest with fibromyalgia symptoms. It's as if the nervous system has blown a fuse. Just like when you blow a fuse at home, someone has to flip the breaker to get the power working again. With Fibro, I've found when patients take some time and space away from the craziness, they can recalibrate their point of view. Time away from the normal routine allows the mind to clear and see things as they really are.

One therapist told my client, "You always have the choice to leave." My client was committed to the 'until death do you part' part of her marriage vows. Her vows had meaning. Leaving wasn't an option. The therapist assured her this wasn't any compromise. In fact, until she acknowledged she had the choice to leave, she never really had the choice to stay. She was making a choice. It was her choice. She could stay or leave. She was stronger by realizing she was making the choice. Whether she decided to stay or leave, it's *her* choice.

When you recognize you can make the choice, the nervous system can calm down. Your primal instincts can relax as that survival part of us realizes you aren't going to suffer endlessly. There is a subtle but strong shift. Choices represent a powerful shift on the road of the healing journey.

Cautionary Tale: You Aren't Crazy

If you have been diagnosed with fibromyalgia, I feel your frustration. As you have been learning, in real life sometimes the only way to deal with it is to go through it. And if you have been diagnosed with fibro, you have already been going through it. You may already be handling multiple appointments with doctors. You may have endured people you love who think you are overreacting and exaggerating or faking your fatigue. Some friends or family may have asked if this could be all in your head. Many people with fibromyalgia question themselves, "Am I imagining my symptoms?"

You are not making this up. The clients I've worked with have told me stories that despite their will to march on, they end up curled into a ball on the bed at 3 pm, sleeping for hours. You are not imagining your symptoms. But it is normal to wonder. It's almost impossible to think straight when you are in pain. Your doctor wants to help, but even the good docs only have so many tools in the toolbox. Some doctors default to prescribing meds.

A word of warning. It's pretty normal for doctors to prescribe antidepressants for fibro. Many patients are depressed because they are in pain. The drugs don't treat the pain. Take a look at the side effects of antidepressants as described by the Mayo Clinic website.[44] These medicines can cause serious additional problems.

Mila hurt all over. Add all the possible side effects from prescription medicine, not a great option for someone already in pain. It's less than ideal for someone already feeling down. Fibromyalgia is a condition that demands we look beyond the physical, beyond biology, to the mental and emotional stress that is often at the heart of the symptoms. We are learning to look for more natural ways to heal.

An option to consider to begin treating fibro is to schedule a session for massage therapy. In 8 out of 10 cases, clients reported feeling a better overall sense of wellness, better mood, and reduced pain. Massage therapy allows a person time to reflect and rest. This calms the nervous system. If sleep is a challenge, massage can help a person fall asleep more quickly and sleep more deeply on the days they get a massage. Research tells us massage treatments help flip the switch from fight or flight (sympathetic nervous system) to rest and digest (parasympathetic nervous system) in over 90% of people with fibromyalgia.

If you are dealing with fibromyalgia, there is a high probability that your pain is a messenger. God bless you for the life lessons you are learning. You may ask, "What am I learning from being in pain?" Fair question.

Some classic lessons my clients have embraced are: What needs to shift? Are you learning how to take care of yourself? Are you learning how to prioritize yourself? Learning how to put yourself first in your relationships? Learning how to put yourself first in your family? *Your* needs are a priority, too. I suggest you are learning that you are worthy. You are enough. You deserve happiness. You are not just the glue that holds the family together. You have a voice. You matter.

⌁ The Exercise: Get Help ⌁

Here's where I'd normally give you an exercise to understand your situation a little better. However, fibromyalgia is not a condition to wrestle with alone. Don't be afraid to seek out professional help. There could be mental and emotional wounds of the past (or present) setting off alarms all over your body. If you don't already have a resource, it could be as easy as a Google search, *mental health near me.*

If you don't think you can afford therapy, who do you know who can give you a referral to a therapist who offers free sessions and/or drastically reduced fees?

Addressing our mental health is as normal as flossing your teeth. You are to be congratulated. If you feel any negative way about exploring your mental health, there is a good chance *someone else* is telling their story to you.

Fibromyalgia is caused in part by a frazzled nervous system. Give your nervous system a break: They can be quiet for now.

No matter what action you choose, speak out loud "I am unique. I am brilliant. I am strong. I am light."

A Final Thought

When it comes to fibromyalgia, no two people are the same. When I met Hanna, I'd seen that look before: Ashamed, startled, yet hopeful. Her eyes lit up the moment she felt heard. It felt like *she mattered* for the first time in a long time. Fibromyalgia is a very serious condition, and *it's very personal.*

If you are in an abusive relationship right now, you can call the Domestic Abuse hotline at 800-799-7233.

Sometimes, talking through the problem out loud can be an amazing relief. Words are powerful and, many times, are the beginning of the healing path.

Today, right where you are, you are on a good path. Continue to follow your heart. This all happens for a reason.

Know that I hold you in the Love and Light of the Universe. I believe in you. You will find your way.

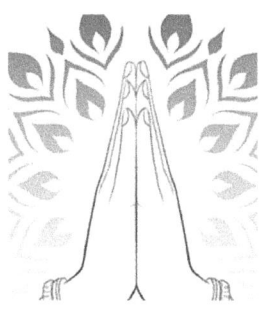

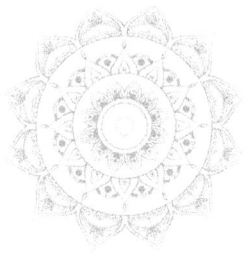

PHANTOM PAIN

*Energy cannot be created or destroyed, it can only
be changed from one form to another.*

~ Albert Einstein

WWII War Hero - Jim

On April 20, 1945, Jim Vining put a sock and a shoe on his right foot for the last time. That same day he climbed into a Martin B26 Marauder to pilot his last flight of World War II. Jim has had phantom pain in that right foot for over 50 years.

It was the summer of 2002 when I met Jim. He was 77 years old and was having his first massage. To be accurate, we met when I was doing seated massages at a local grocery store. I was there promoting my massage business. Jim decided that he liked the 15 minutes so much he'd sign up for an hour.

When he arrived at the office, I asked if he had any injuries he wanted to let me know about. He just smiled a big ol' Cheshire Cat smile. As a man who had lived almost his whole life with half a leg, Jim had a story to tell. He answered, "I've had a few injuries." He explained his primary concern was that he had had phantom pain in his *missing* right foot for his entire adult life. He was curious if massage could help. I asked what his phantom pain felt like? He says it feels like stepping onto hot tar with the bottom of his foot coming off.

For those who know their WWII history, the combat was basically over by April 1945, but that day, someone forgot to tell the Germans. Jim's plane was hit by enemy fire and badly damaged. After the explosion rocked his plane, Jim stared down at where his lower leg used to be. He was losing blood. His right lower leg and foot had been blown off just below the knee. Minutes mattered. The plane crash-landed. The co-pilot radioed for help. One of his crew was dead. By the grace of God, Allied support arrived quickly.

While he waited for their arrival, he held a tight grip on the stump to stop his bleeding. He winced as he told me the story of how his crew member twisted fabric into a makeshift tourniquet. He and his crewmates were put in the back of a pickup truck. Jim passed out bouncing down a country road in Germany with no idea if he would even survive the injury.

When he opened his eyes, he was lying in a hospital bed in France. The lower half of his right leg had been amputated below the knee. He told me he felt lucky because the doctors saved his knee. "Life would have been more difficult without a knee. I wouldn't have been able to ride a bike." Jim was awarded the Silver Star for bravery. I believe courage was one of the themes of Jim's life.

The Treatment

He asked if, during the massage, I would treat the end of his stump. I was surprised at his request. With some amputees, the stump is an area to avoid. Quite the contrary, Jim identified this area as the source of his phantom pain and wondered if the massage could help. I said of course I'd do my best. This was Jim's first massage and my first amputee client. It was a new experience for both of us. My job was to use my professional training, do what I knew how to do, and trust the process. I was nervous before entering the treatment room. I set the intention to facilitate a space for his body to heal as much as it was ready to heal. I thought to myself, *This should be interesting*.

One of the first things I noticed as I entered the treatment room was that Jim's prosthetic leg was propped up in the corner. Working on an amputee feels oddly intimate. Like it could be a violation of privacy. Depending on the person, a stump may be a do not touch, do not talk too much about, closed subject, no-go zone. I gave myself a little pep talk. *I'm well qualified. I've been invited to do the work. I've been asked to help. No pressure. The worst-case scenario is that the rest of Jim's body feels better.* I wondered and hoped that the massage would help with his chronic phantom pain.

Sometimes old wounds hold old memories. The memories are stored in the muscles like a snapshot in time. A Polaroid picture layered within the emotions. As the muscle relaxes, it can release memories from a specific place and time. These muscle memories can create feelings. We talked about Muscle Memory in the introduction. As I laid my hands on Jim's body, I acknowledged it as sacred ground. It always is, but this time I could be stepping into an unmarked minefield of old wounds. I proceeded with caution and care.

Jim's massages treated his body head to toe, but I would spend extra time on his residual limb. As I massaged the stump, I felt the callouses that had built up over the years as the leg had rubbed against his prosthetic.

Later in our experience together, he would tell me about his first prosthetic. He got it before being discharged from the hospital. It was whittled from wood around 1945. That rudimentary peg leg gave him mobility but also numbness, splinters, and wounds on the end of his tender stump.

During that first massage, I felt the tissue start to loosen, and I became keenly aware that the nerve bundles of his missing lower leg and foot were just below the surface of my fingers. I needed to be very kind. In my mind, I spoke to the stump and missing limb. I thanked the body for its sacrifice. I invited the gnarled nerves to unwind. My intuition guided me to do energy work on the missing lower leg and foot. With one hand on the physical knee and the other hand cupping the invisible foot, I visualized cool, clear water pouring over the fiery heat on the bottom of the missing foot. I imagined the foot dipping into chilly ocean water. I imagined restoring balance.

As providence would have it, after the massage, the phantom pain would release its grip for three, four, sometimes even five days. That was a victory for both of us. Jim and I worked together for a decade. He was a humble, grateful, and dedicated warrior for peace. He was a true hero on many levels. He was brave to explore the benefits of massage in his 70s. He passed away peacefully at 92 years old, joining his beloved wife of over 50 years, Mary Frances. A life well lived. I've included -with permission-a personal recount in Jim's own words in Appendix I. Peace to you, Jim Vining. March 14, 1925 - August 8, 2017.

The Lesson: What is Your Superpower?

Could your weakness really be your superpower? Some think of being an amputee as a disadvantage. Certainly, none of us would choose to lose a limb. However, Jim turned this tragedy into triumph. Jim volunteered at events to tell the story of his WWII experiences. He was a bold advocate for peace, and people really listened and considered his point of view. He had sacrificed a limb.

But Jim also had a great sense of humor. One such story I had never heard was shared with me by his daughter, Bonnie. During a big rainy downpour, Jim was leaving work at the Pentagon. He was holding his umbrella in one hand, ready to open it as soon as he got outside. The other hand pushed the glass of the revolving door. A guardsman hollered, "Goodnight!" as Jim exited. As Jim looked back over his shoulder to respond, his umbrella (brolly) got caught in the door. Jim lost his balance, and his ankle got caught in the revolving door. He lurched to avoid falling when something abruptly stopped the door. To the horror of the guardsman, Jim's leg was in the revolving door. His colleague didn't realize Jim had a prosthetic. His leg had come off in the tussle and Jim had been propelled on his one good leg out the door and into the rain. Pale as a ghost, the guardsman rushed to help thinking there had been an accident. Jim saw what happened, and hopped on one leg, but couldn't get back into the revolving door fast enough to tell the co-worker he wasn't injured. A moment later, his comrade realized what happened and felt relieved and ridiculous. They both laughed when the vigilant sentinel said he was very happy Jim had a prosthetic leg.

Over the twelve years I worked with Jim, I have to admit I was disappointed that the phantom pain never totally went away.

Massage gave him temporary relief, but I had hoped for more. Thomas Edison said, "I have not failed. I have just found 10,000 ways that did not work." The lesson for me has been that in my weakness, I can find my superpower. Tackling a new challenge means there's going to have to be a new answer. I was open and willing to find those answers. Even if the outcome didn't look like I thought it should. My weakness of not knowing the perfect technique allowed me to explore, research, *and accept* that what I was doing was good enough. I may have expected more, but it was more than Jim expected.

In many ways, Jim inspired me to regularly practice stretching outside of my comfort zone. He lost his lower right leg when he was 20. That could have been his story for the rest of his life. He knew he had a choice to make. His entire life could be about his disability or his ability. He could have chosen bitterness. He wanted to use his story to demonstrate and advocate that there should never be another war. If losing his leg would stir emotion within people, he was determined to use that stirring to plead for peace.

⌒ The Exercise: Shifting From Drama to Empowerment ⌒

What's *your* weakness? What is your phantom pain? Is it physical? Is it mental? Is it emotional? Maybe a bit of all three?

Pain isn't always physical. Pain can be emotional. Are you telling a victim story about how you grew up? Pain can be mental. Do you regularly feel the need to step in and rescue someone from bad decisions because you're worried about them? Sometimes pain shows up in our emotions. Are you pissed off for a really good reason? In the workshop taught by Greg Coles, "Making the Shift from Drama to Empowerment" he addresses the roles of the Victim, the Rescuer, and the Persecutor. This "Drama Triangle" was first described by Stephen Karpman, MD in 1968. And it leads us to a shift into the Empowerment Dynamic.

David Emerald and Donna Zajonic have been teaching this work for over a decade all over the world. I have adapted an exercise from The Empowerment Dynamic to help you transform your weakness(es) into your superpower.

Please thoughtfully answer these questions:

1. Who are the victims I know?
2. Who are rescuers I know?
3. Who are persecutors I know?

Which role do you resonate with the most?

- Victim
- Rescuer
- Persecutor

Think of one person you are in this role with regularly.

How could you move from:

Victim   → to → Creator?

Rescuer   → to → Coach?

Persecutor → to → Challenger?

CAUTION: Ask permission to coach. We must ask permission to offer our point of view. One way would be saying something like, "Would you be willing to consider looking at this situation in a different way?"

Maybe your weakness is more tangible. Are you scared of public speaking, or spiders, or small crowded spaces? How could that be a superpower? Would you be willing to consider looking at this situation in a different way? The good doctor Susan Jeffers says, "Feel the fear and do it anyway." When you name it, you claim it. It's easier to tame it. Release the shame of it. Even make a game of it. Just by identifying the thing you call a weakness, your readiness to release it grows.

Remember, you are perfect just the way you are. It's true! And your weakness is part of your perfection.

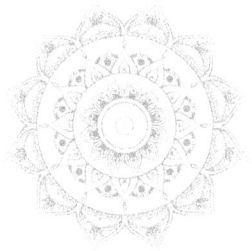

CONCLUSION

Do what you feel in your heart to be right,
for you will be criticized anyway.

~ Eleanor Roosevelt

What a journey you, dear reader, have been on. We are here together, you and I, by divine order. I believe you were meant to read this book. You were destined to find this information. Someone upstairs is looking out for you. That's pretty cool.

So, now what?

Pause. Take a big, deep breath of beautiful air and allow a smile to curl the ends of your mouth. Now you have some answers! Now you have the opportunity to take a very important next step. Practice radical kindness. What is radical kindness? It is committing, promising, and doing the very best you can do to be boldly kind. And, my lovely, here's the hard part: For this to work, *you must start by being radically kind to yourself.* Yes.

Be radically kind to yourself.

1. Reward yourself. Rewards can be a simple pleasure - such as watching the sunset with your favorite beverage, taking an afternoon nap, writing with a great pen, buying yourself flowers, and arranging them in a new Goodwill vase. Staring at the ocean, window shopping, stomping in a puddle, riding your bike in the rain. There are so many simple pleasures.

2. Change negative self-talk right now. Our inner dialogue is critical to our healing journey. We can catch ourselves telling lies like:

   I have bad genes. No, you don't.

   Or, *I'm a mess.* No, you are not. You are perfect just the way you are.

   I can never fully recover from this. Yes, you can. It just doesn't seem that way right now.

   I have a bad shoulder (knee, hip). No, you don't. You have pain in your shoulder. Or your knee. Or in your hip.

   Work with me here. If you have a body part not cooperating, say it out loud,

   "My _____ needs more attention."

   "My _____ is still getting back to 100%."

   "My _____ reminds me to be more cautious when I _____."

Let go of the old dialogue and *replace it with intentional new phrases.* Get specific. Perhaps the phrase "All is well," covers a multitude of situations, but challenge yourself to be specific: My shoulder is healing. My knee is getting stronger. My lower back is stable, solid, and balanced.

Positive internal dialogue lifts your spirits and can make you feel better. Do you have some inaccurate beliefs about yourself? Often, we don't know. In the past, have you been told things like:

"You're such a mess."
"You always screw things up."
"You have never really been college material."

Just pull those old labels off. Put the labels, criticisms, and negative comments in an imaginary box. They aren't the truth of who you are. Put a lid on that box and walk it out the front door.

Now you get to replace the old inaccurate labels with new, true labels that work for you. Fill in the blank:

I'm really good at _____.
I am a _____ person. (generous, kind, friendly)
My last big/little win was when I _____.

How are you feeling? Emotions play a big role in motivation. Positive labels create positive feelings. Yay, you! This leads to the next and possibly most important guideline.

Forgive, forgive, forgive. Forgive everyone all the time, but especially yourself. This is a principle I'm taking directly from the book, *The Four Spiritual Laws of Prosperity* by Edwene Gaines.[45] Others also endorse forgiveness as a means to a more peaceful life. Who do you need to forgive? No one? Then focus on forgiving yourself. Would you say this out loud? "I love and accept myself exactly the way I am." Repeat three times.

Once you embrace the idea of viewing your body's pain and disease as offering you a message, I believe you will be able to live your truth more fully. In doing so, you are shining your light. I share with you the beautiful words of Marianne Williamson, "As we let our own light shine, we unconsciously give other people permission to do the same."[46]

The Spirit in me beholds the Spirit in you.

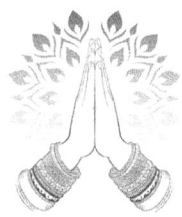

APPENDIX I

JIM VINING'S
WWII EXPERIENCE
IN A MARTIN B-26 MARAUDER

For gallantry in action against the enemy in aerial flight.
On 20 April 1945, Lt. Vining, serving as pilot of a B-26
type aircraft during an attack over enemy marshalling yards
in the area of Mimmingen, Germany, distinguished himself by
heroic devotion to duty and exceptional courage. While over
the target area, his flight was attacked by a numerically
superior force of enemy fighters. Although his aircraft was
severely damaged and he himself critically injured, Lt.
Vining refused to withdraw from the flight. Determinedly
holding his position he directed a brilliant attack against
the enemy planes, while his gunners destroyed two. Only
after his flight had dropped their bomb load upon the enemy
target did Lt. Vining accept first aid. The superior aerial
skill and leadership evidenced by Lt. Vining on this occasion
reflect great credit upon himself and are in keeping with the
finest traditions of the Army Air Forces.

This citation from General Order No. 158, Headquarters 9th
Air Force, 11 August 1945, for the SILVER STAR award is manifestly
typical, in its distorted data and platitudinous puffery, of some
rear-echelon functionaries' proclivity to gloss, misconstrue and
misrepresent the essentially horrendous elements of a combat
calamity; which may, incidentally, explain why the recommendation
for the MEDAL OF HONOR (written by our Intelligence Officer - a
man of integrity and deep sensitivity - who went to extraordinary
lengths to obtain the complete story) was ignored. I have never
become embittered by such wholesale evidence of human turpitude; I
only wish to record for the sake of accurate history and perhaps
an appreciative posterity the true account of what happened that
day to me and an exceptionally devoted and courageous crew whose
performance placed them forever among the nation's unsung heroes.

It offers a textbook study of a day of paradoxical irony.
The "Stars and Stripes" headline on the previous day (AIR WAR IS
OVER) had rekindled the sometimes flagging hope of ultimately
surviving combat. Also, having flown the last previous mission
a couple of days earlier - a milk run to the same area - we should
not have been scheduled for the mission on the 20th. However,
despite the good news and Patton's arrival in Czechoslovakia, the
inimitable "powers that be" decided on an "all out effort,"
requiring every available plane that could possibly be airborne.
Thus was my crew scheduled for this unnecessary strike. Following
a routine briefing, during which Intelligence confirmed that all
German aerial resistance had collapsed, an eventuality developed
which - in retrospect - seemed to presage the ultimate trajedy
that at the moment appeared so remote. Due to a shortage of
planes in our squadron, and in order for us to provide a
proportionate share of crews, a sister squadron "loaned" us the
ship assigned to my crew. It was a standard, if macabre, jest
that a borrowed plane was usually the worst in the lender's
inventory. Among the numerous defects gradually discovered in
this particular junkyard fugitive, the immediate and most critical
was a malfunctioning bomb release!

But the hard-pressed ground crew succeeded in rectifying the problem, allowing us to start engines, about one half hour past our scheduled takeoff time. So, instead of being third, ours was the last of 48 planes to depart; thus it was theoretically impossible, considering the geometrically complex procedures prescribed, for us to attain our designated position in the formation. Nevertheless, in addition to having long since mastered all the demanding techniques of B-26 flying, I had developed some personal, unorthodox methods to cope with just this kind of emergency. All judgments to-the-contrary-notwithstanding we successfully joined the formation prior to penetrating enemy territory.

The next disconcerting incident ensued shortly after we had joined up and crossed the Rhine into southern Germany. A brief but heavy display of flak bursts suddenly erupted throughout the formation over a valley where no recent sighting of AAA batteries had been observed. Always unnerving, these encounters no longer generated the deep anxiety characteristic of the early combat sorties. This was my fortieth. Of that total only four or five had been milk runs. We had consistently returned to base with varying degrees of flak damage; resulting, on several occasions, in critical emergency landings but never with personal injuries. Consequently, I had assumed the rather fatalistic attitude that I would never be shot down by flak; a sound intuition that afforded only a small degree of consolation at the end.

In time we arrived over Kempten, the target two days earlier, which served as the I.P. (Initial Point for beginning a bomb run) for this day's target at Memmingen. The order of battle for this mission required each of the eight flights to approach the target in succession. Mine was last in line and, as we executed a sharp left turn over Kempten, our growing complacency was abruptly shattered by the simultaneous appearance of small calibre flak bursts and an alarming number of Me-262, jet fighters. The surprising advent of the jets was signalled via the inter-com by engineer/tail gunner, Yates, who commenced firing at the first one as they approached from the rear in single file. At almost incredible speed the jet passed over the center planes in our flight barely high enough to avoid a rear-end collision with the flight leader. The second, a few seconds behind, was even nearer a collision course.

As time seemed suspended, lending an unreal, slow-motion cast to this frightening scene, the third jet appeared off my left wing and barely clearing our number four plane by inches. In that timeless interval I knew that he could not avoid colliding with our number one plane. Clearly desperate, shoving his stick forward in an attempt to pass under, he left most of his vertical stabilizer behind; chewed up by the right propellor of our leader. Apparently due to some loss of control he drifted to the right instead of performing a customary post strike left turn. This placed him directly in line of fire not only from the bombardier's 50 calibre gun but from four others, fixed two on each side of the

fuselage primarily for ground strafing purposes; a type of attack
no longer attempted by B-26s at that late date. Most pilots
disregarded these guns while my own sense of orderliness required
that all guns to be cleaned and charged prior to a mission. So,
with a perfect target dead ahead I automatically pressed the
firing button on the control wheel while turning slightly to the
right to move the tracer pattern from the rear of the jet toward
the cockpit and engines. But he was also losing altitude which
would require me to nose down to finish the job. With extreme
reluctance I ceased firing and moved back into formation in
deference to sound defensive doctrine and disciplined training.

On closing my position as tightly as possible on our number
four plane I glanced quickly over my left shoulder to confirm a
terrible suspicion that a fourth jet was reaching his firing
position behind us. In the next instant, as I double-checked my
position, a stunning blast thrust me from the controls and the
plane rolled sharply to the right due to loss of power in the
starboard engine.

Although my memory of the details of that incident is as
clear-cut and distinct today as it was in the days immediately
following the next 100 seconds after the detonation of the 30mm
shell have always been essentially impossible to articulate in a
sequential, comprehensive narrative. Myriad decisions, emotions,
impressions, judgments and questions coursed concurrently through
my conciousness. This awesome activity, which could only be
characterized as "superhuman," prompted some dexterous responses
to the crisis. Sensing that my right foot had been severed above
the ankle, I instantly directed co-pilot, Mulvihill, to take his
controls while I moved in swift succession to feather the right
propellor, crank left turn into the rudder trim tab, and signal
the bombardier, Wells, to jettison the bomb load. Until that
moment we had been losing altitude at a rate of 2000 feet per
minute; we had been hit 4000 feet above the mountains. The
remainder of the flight was already miles away and for a few
agonizing seconds we were alone. (So much for refusing to
withdraw from the flight and bombing the target; the flight
withdrew from me)

Suddenly we were the center of attention of a plethora of
jets, arriving from all directions. Abandoning their previous
procedure of attack, and possibly assuming that we were now an
easy kill, quickly cost them four aircraft at the hands of my
determined gunners. As they later recalled, "it was like shooting
fish in a barrel."

The shooting was over, temporarily, within 10 minutes of the
initial attack but we were still in dire peril of crashing in
forbidding terrain. However, the receding elevation coupled with
a gradual decrease in our rate of descent created a glimmer of
hope that we could escape. At least that became my plan for my
crew and plane; for myself I was under no illusion that I could
survive. Some two to three minutes after the initial trauma, in

the infinitesimal lull before the second attack, I got a quick
glance at my severed leg. The main artery was hosing the
remaining blood in my body into a deepening, coagulating pool
already covering most of the flight deck. Assuming it was too
late I nonetheless clamped both hands above the knee and with the
superhuman strength of pumping adrenalin I was able to slow the
flow to a trickle; maintaining this posture throughout the ensuing
fight.

    For a half hour, with some obvious interruptions, after he
took control of the plane I delivered an oral manual on emergency
operation of the B-26 to Mulvihill. I did not repeat a single
instruction, nor did he forget any. A severe handicap to
operating the plane from the right seat was the absence of brake
pedals which added to the hazard of a single-engine landing on a
runway if he were fortunate enough to reach one. Another serious
complication lay in the fact that to allow the bombardier to exit
the nose section the co-pilot was required to slide his seat aft
about three feet to clear a passage way. After dropping the bombs
Wells' had asked whether I could get him out of the nose. I had
replied in the affirmative. As will be subsequently described
this did occur but only barely saving his life. For three weeks
following the fateful crash Wells was not expected to survive.
During that period, while able to speak only in a weakened
whisper, he insisted on relating the details of the exit to the
squadron intelligence officer whose response was previously noted.
As an ancient seer observed, "truth is [indeed] stranger than
fiction."

    Upon leaving the target area I had directed Mulvihill to
follow a northwesterly heading that would take us across the front
lines at Stuttgart, rather than the westerly return that would
lead to another encounter with the lately located flak batteries.
Termination of the jet attacks allowed me to call radio operator/
gunner, Armstrong, forward render first aid. He swiftly applied a
tourniquet which freed my left hand for other tasks during the
remainder of the flight. My seating position precluded applying
sulfa powder to the injury site. Then we discovered another
defect of a "borrowed" plane - the water thermos had not been
filled. Without water chewing a sulfa tablet was an unpleasant
exercise in futility. I refused the last assistance available
from the first aid kit - a shot of morphine which I erroneously
thought would produce instant sleep. Also, my only discomfort was
a painfully dry throat which had developed at the moment of trauma
indicating a rapid loss of blood.

    No sooner were these limited ministrations complete when the
voice of Yates broke the silence with the announcement that more
jets were closing from the rear. Aware that we could not survive
another attack if the jets obviously were resuming their standard
procedure I elected evasive action, much as we routinely countered
flak attacks (which I had already judged could have saved us from
harm in the first place had the flight leader thought of it), and
it worked like a charm. Considering that their standard firing

run terminated with a break to the left we were left with one unhappy choice - a quick right turn of about 10 degrees. But a turn into a dead engine required a higher airspeed which could only be gained by a slight dive with a loss of precious altitude. Mulvihill momentarily demurred at this suggestion but quickly understood the truth of the matter; if we were forced all the way to the ground it would be better to go in with one engine still running. I also knew that Yates would fire first so when I heard his guns I signalled for the right turn which was executed three times in quick succession as three jets swept harmlessly past our left wing while I thumbed my nose at each pilot.

The reaction of the third jet pilot was startling. With a look of sheer panic he violently nosed down, diving straight for the ground. Curious, I looked behind him and was more amazed to see two P-51s who had gained on him while he slowed down to attack us. About a half mile behind when he nosed down the P-51s rolled over in perfect formation and, flying inverted, cut the jet off in his dive and forced him straight into the ground. That was the only help we had that day; thereafter we were alone in the sky.

Passing over Stuttgart some 30 minutes after the initial attack I resisted a strong impulse and the urging of the crew to land at the large airfield there. According to the intelligence briefing that morning this field had been the objective of our ground forces the day before; therefore, we could not be sure who controlled it at 1130 on the 20th. By this time I had completed the instruction list and all contingencies were planned for. With nothing more to occupy my immediate attention I began to assess my personal condition, wondering if death would occur suddenly. Apparent fatigue and a growing throbbing sensation in my leg indicated that I should relax and relinquish complete command to Mulvihill. I allowed the morphine to be injected only to be chagrined that it did not put me to sleep. To further relax I discarded earphones and throat mike, becoming incommunicado, and kept an eye on the engine instruments so that I would be the first to detect its inevitable failure in another 30 minutes.

At the end of what seemed to me now in a growing euphoria to be another five to ten minute interval Mulvihill executed a 360 degree left turn. Thinking he was making a course correction which, but for the dead engine, would have been a short turn to the right I did not question him until he started to repeat the circle. He did not tell me that another 30 minutes had passed but did say that he and Wells had determined that we could not reach Trier and the nearest large airport. Therefore he was initiating one of the options that I had given in my instructions, i.e., selecting a town where medical assistance might be available and making a belly landing in an open field as near the town as possible. We circling such a town (unknown to me to this day) and I reminded him that Wells must exit the nose. Reluctantly, he yielded the controls to me for the last time while, with remaining foot and free left hand, I continued the left-banked two-minute turn which permitted Wells to crawl aft to join Armstrong in the

navigator/radio compartment. Then, for the next two minutes, with
Yates having come forward and kneeling between us to handle the
engine controls Mulvihill established a landing pattern into what
appeared to be a perfectly suitable wheat field.

As we turned on final approach, less than three minutes since
I had flown the plane, I was sharply alerted by an alarm signal
deep in my brain which, undetected by me, had been slipping into
unconsciousness. A swift perusal of instruments, controls and
crew revealed nothing amiss so I looked over the nose at the
approaching ground. At about 75 feet above the ground I stared in
utter horror at what had been invisible (due to clever camouflage)
until that instant - a yawning tank trap stretching across the
field at the very point of touchdown. With no time to utter a
word and almost by sheer instinct I grasped my wheel to pull the
nose up into a stall and half-spin into the ground; instantly
calculating that half of us might survive when no one could
possibly do so if we hit the ditch nose first at 150 mph. But the
exertion of reaching for the wheel consumed my last gram of energy
and coma finally rendered me<u>hors de combat.</u>

About 10 minutes later I awoke to find myself on a litter
stretched across the back of a jeep, held in place by a soldier at
each end. While the driver got us under way these men assured me
that we had landed safely (I didn't learn the grim truth about the
fatal crash until three months had passed), my crew was safe, and
I was being transported to a general hospital in Metz, France.
With two more very brief moments of consciousness, I knew almost
nothing of that three and a half hour trip except that each time I
was told that my crew was alright. It is still painful to recall
that I was finally informed of the death in the crash of armorer/
gunner, Winger, by his parents who for over two months had only
been informed that he was "missing in action!" Winger died alone,
having been obliged to remain in the tail section as a lookout.
In addition to Wells, Armstrong had been seriously injured. Only
Mulvihill and Yates had been able to extricate themselves from the
wreckage, though both were painfully bruised. I was limp and
sustained no further injury.

Pictures of the scene, taken two weeks later and officially
sent to me by an investigating team (presumably I was cleared of
any responsibility for losing the plane), still cause me to
experience profound wonder that anyone survived. Considerable
credit must be given to a much much maligned airplane that
protected its crews far better than any other plane in WWII. My
progress from trauma through coma to the very abyss of death and
beyond to an entirely new life can only be described, perhaps
inadequately, as miraculous, but that is another chapter....

Wells received emergency treatment from the German physician
we were seeking for me. He was fully credited by American doctors
for saving Wells' life, though it hung in the balance for a time.
Without blood or plasma nothing could be done for me at the scene;
hence the long trek to Metz which placed me in the care of

excellent surgeons and nurses in a hospital that was named for me as long as it was in that location. Both Wells and Armstrong fully recovered to return to normal, productive lives as did Mulvihill and Yates. I enjoyed the warm friendship of Winger's aging parents for the remaining years of their lives. Wells (who had been the oldest member of the crew at 33; I was youngest at 20) died at age 67 after a series of strokes. Four of us are aging, if not to perfection, to a fine vintage.

My own life continues to be an exciting pilgrimage under the auspices of the Divine Being who created everything. Its finest hours - not only those now rare ones when I am on a solo flight - are best limned by my favorite poem, composed by another young pilot who met an untimely death, entitled HIGH FLIGHT

Oh! I have slipped the surly bonds of earth,
    And danced the skies on laughter-silvered wings;
Sunward I've climbed and joined the tumbling mirth
    Of sun-split clouds - and done a hundred things
You have not dreamed of - wheeled and soared and swung
    High in the sunlit silence, hov'ring there
I've chased the shouting wind along
    And flung my eager craft through footless of air.
Up, up the long delirious burning blue
    I've topped the windswept heights with easy grace
Where never lark, or even eagle flew
    And, while with silent, lifting mind I've trod
The high untrespassed sanctity of space,
    Put out my hand, and touched the face of God.

John Gillespie Magee, Jr.

Valor

By John L. Frisbee, Contributing Editor

Beating the Luftwaffe's Best

How a B-26 straggler, its pilot critically wounded, survived repeated attacks by Luftwaffe jet fighters.

APRIL 20, 1945, promised to be a good day for twenty-year-old 1st Lt. Jim Vining, a B-26 aircraft commander of the 323d Bomb Group based at Valenciennes in northern France. The forty-eight crews that were to bomb marshaling yards at Memmingen in southwest Germany had been briefed to expect no opposition from Luftwaffe fighters and little if any flak. Allied armies were closing in on Berlin; German surrender could be only days away.

Lieutenant Vining had flown his thirty-ninth mission—a milk run—the previous day. Today's strike had the earmarks of another. He could not know that he was to become the central character in one of the most unusual but little-noted dramas of World War II.

Jim Vining was assigned a war-weary B-26 borrowed from another squadron. By the time it was ready to roll, the bomber stream had disappeared to the southeast. He would have been justified in aborting, but that wasn't Vining's style. At max cruise, he caught up with the formation as it crossed the Rhine. There, the benign operational briefing began to break down. The bombers were greeted by heavy flak. When they turned north at Kempten on a bomb run to Memmingen, they were attacked by some twenty Me-262 jet fighters, each armed with four 30-mm cannon firing explosive shells.

Three of the German jets attacked Vining's flight leader, the third coming so close that part of its tail was chewed off by the flight leader's right propeller. As the -262 flashed past Vining, he broke from formation and opened fire with his four forward-firing .50-caliber guns, scoring hits before the jet dove away. Vining pulled back into formation and immediately was hit by a fourth -262 that had come up from behind. The Lieutenant felt what he describes as "a

slight sting" in his leg. Looking down, he saw his right foot dangling by a shred of skin, blood gushing from the severed artery. Simultaneously, the right engine went to idle, and the B-26 rolled sharply to the right.

Before attempting to stanch the flow of blood from his severed foot, Vining helped his copilot, Lt. Jim Mulvihill, roll the wings level. He then feathered the right prop, trimmed the plane for one-engine flight, and signaled the bombardier to jettison the bomb load. Only then did Vining use both hands to compress the pressure point behind his right leg to slow the flow of blood.

Now a straggler, Vining's B-26 was attacked by several Me-262s coming in from all directions and turning violently to avoid each other. Though gradually weakening from shock and loss of blood, he continued to act as aircraft commander, telling his copilot when to break to spoil the enemy attacks and drive them away.

Ten minutes later, three enemy jets returned. Vining continued to direct his crew's defense. Thanks to his split-second tactical assessments, the jets scored no hits on the B-26. During the two engagements in which his gunners believed they shot down four -262s, Vining gave his copilot, who had come to the group directly from pilot training with no B-26 transition, a cram course on how to get the bomber safely on the ground.

Vining did not believe he would survive, but he was determined to save the crew. He told them to set course for Trier, the nearest field that could handle a single-engine landing flown by a copilot whose controls did not have brake pedals.

During its engagements with the -262s, the B-26 had been forced down to less than 3,000 feet. When the last of the enemy fighters left and waist gunner TSgt. N. C. Armstrong had applied a tourniquet to Lieutenant Vining's leg, they were near Stuttgart. Vining knew they could not clear the mountains bordering the Rhine. The crew refused to bail out and leave him to die in the inevitable crash. He told copilot

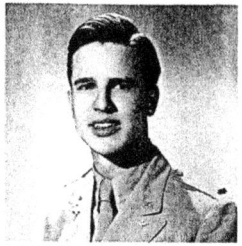

Despite severe injuries, Jim Vining tried to save his crew.

Mulvihill to find a suitable field and prepare to belly in, but first bombardier SSgt. J. D. Wells had to get out of the nose. That required the copilot to slide his seat back, out of reach of the controls, to give Wells access to the flight deck.

While that was being done, Vining took control of the B-26 and flew a 360° turn to the left before losing consciousness. The belly landing, with flight engineer TSgt. Paul Yates assisting Mulvihill, would have been successful had it not been for an unobserved tank trap. When the B-26 hit the trap, it broke up, killing the top turret gunner, SSgt. Bill Winger, and critically injuring Wells.

By coincidence, they had landed beside a hospital train whose medics gave them emergency care. Vining, near death from loss of blood, was rushed by Jeep to an Army hospital at Metz, three-and-a-half hours away. Both he and Wells survived.

Lieutenant Vining was awarded the Silver Star for extraordinary heroism that April day fifty years ago. Copilot Mulvihill received the Distinguished Flying Cross. Vining was promoted to captain, retired for physical disability, and completed graduate school. Later, he spent thirty years with the CIA before retiring in the Washington, D. C., area, where he continues to fly. As the saying goes, you can't keep a good man down.   ∎

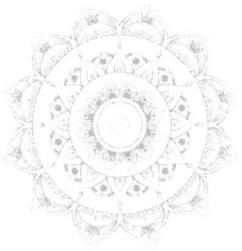

JIM VINING'S OBITUARY

James Louis Vining, Captain USAF (retired), Silver Star decorated veteran, died peacefully on Tuesday, August 8, 2017. James had a life-long love of flying, which led him to enlist in the Army Air Corps at age 18 in 1943. He piloted the B-26 Martin Marauder, and he and his crew flew many successful bombing missions during the war.

On his final mission in the last days of WWII, his plane was struck by a German shell. Despite a life-threatening injury to his right leg, James and his co-pilot managed to successfully land their badly damaged aircraft, losing only one crew member. Due to his injury, James was honorably discharged from the service. After the war, he returned to Louisiana State University, where he finished his BA and MA, married his college sweetheart, [Mary Frances Hodges], and went on to pursue a successful career with the Federal Government.

James was a member and deacon at Vienna Baptist Church for more than 50 years, where he sang in the choir and performed in many dramatic productions. He continued to pursue his love of flying, and after retiring from the government in 1981. He pledged himself to work for peace and a world without war. James loved his family, flying, traveling, and playing games with his grandchildren. He will be greatly missed.

He is warmly remembered.

Namaste.

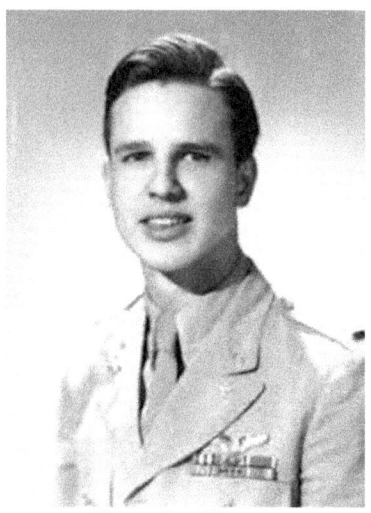
Young Jim Vining

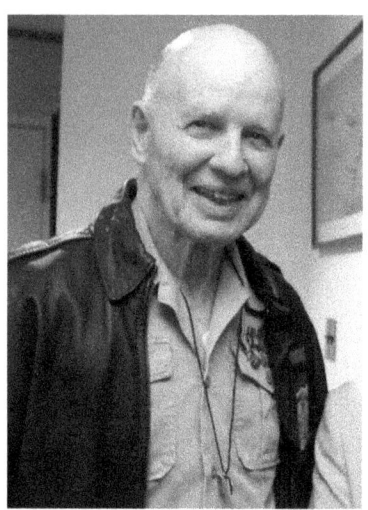
Jim Vining on Veterans Day.

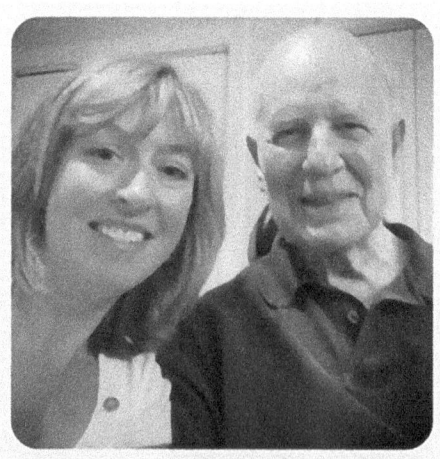
Jodi and Jim

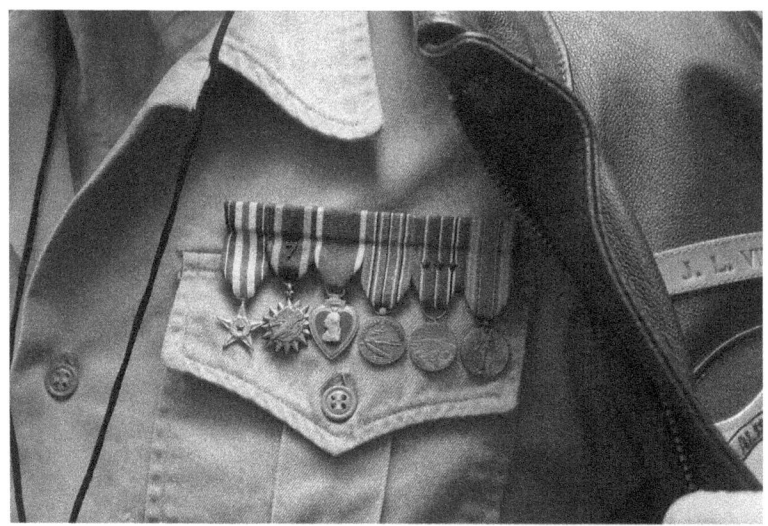

Jim Vining's Medals

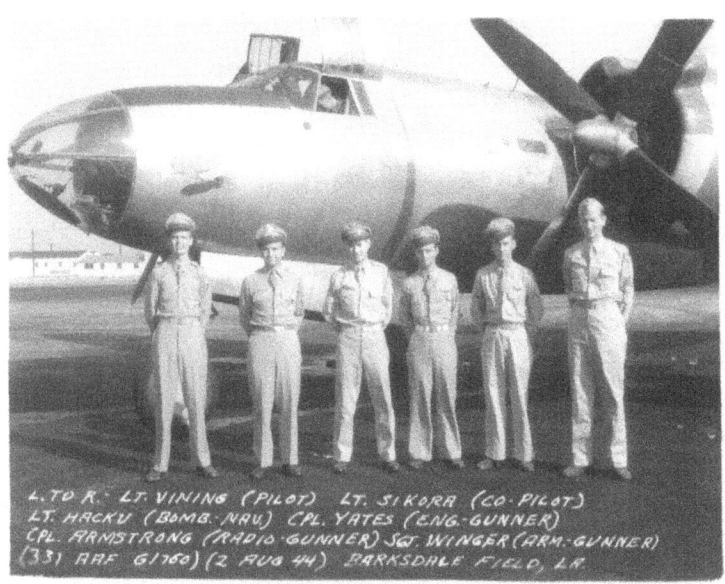

Jim Vining with Crew

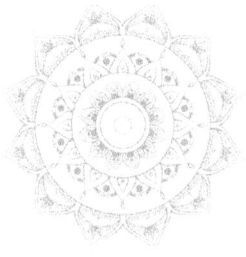

5 COMMON QUESTIONS ABOUT HOW TO EXPERIENCE AN EXCELLENT MASSAGE

1. How do I find a qualified Licensed Massage Therapist?

Use referrals. Ask a friend. Ask the local yoga instructor. Ask a chiropractor for a referral to a Licensed Massage Therapist. Get three recommendations. Of course, you can look online too.

When making the appointment, speak with the actual therapist or to an employee who has gotten a massage from them. In the United States, the correct term for a person who performs massage is *Massage Therapist*. In the United States, the name masseuse/masseur now implies an association with elicit sex trade. Best to use the title, Massage Therapist when making your inquiries. Ask the following questions:

- How long have you been a Licensed Massage Therapist? (LMT) If they answer under a year, move on.

- How would you describe your massage style? Listen to the answer. Does that sound like a good match for you or not so much?
- Do you use a Health Intake Sheet? (answer needs to be yes)
- What are your rates? Give yourself permission to spend $100+ on a massage. This Licensed Healthcare Professional is going to spend over an hour with you.

These questions will give you an idea of the LMT's personal style. If you don't like the vibe, wish them well and let them know you are just gathering information. Then dial the next number.

2. **What can I expect when I arrive?**

You can expect a professional space. One that is clean, organized and inviting. You can expect a Licensed Massage Therapist to be professionally dressed.

You can expect to fill out some paperwork. You may receive a Health Intake form in advance, but you may not. The Massage Therapist will do a thorough health intake prior to the session. From the moment you walk in the office, your information is confidential. Massage Therapists follow Standards of Practice that require they keep your health information and verbal communication confidential.

You can expect your therapist to instruct you on how to lay on the massage table. It is called a massage table. The instructions will be to crawl under the sheet and blanket, like you are getting into bed. You will also be told to lay down either face up or face down. Before getting on the massage table, you will remove some, or all of your clothes. Some clients take off all their clothes. Other clients leave some articles of clothing on. You choose.

If taking off all your clothes doesn't feel comfortable, you can choose to wear your underwear, a one piece bathing suit or a pair of Lycra shorts. It does not matter to the therapist what you take off or leave on. What does matter, what is most important, is that *you* are comfortable.

You can expect that during the massage you will be draped. For example, when massaging your arm, your arm will be out from under the sheet and blanket. The sheet will be securely draped under or around your arm. This is true for your legs, your back also. Breasts, breast tissue, and the pubic region are not exposed at any time.

You can expect to be asked questions during your session. This massage is *your* session. If something doesn't feel good, you have permission to say stop. You have permission to say, "That doesn't feel good." or "That is too much pressure for me."

You can expect to give feedback during the session. An experienced therapist will adjust the pressure or the approach based on your comments. The quality of your customized massage session depends on you using your voice. Massage therapists can tell where the muscles are tight; they can't tell how sore you are. So, your interaction during the massage is critical to designing a session that works best for you.

3. Do I have to have my butt massaged?

No you don't. But you might want to.

Have you ever gone to stand up and your legs and lower back were feeling stiff? You realize, *Oh, I've been sitting for a long time.*

Sitting on your butt 8+ hours a day can decrease circulation and cause stiffness. Sitting also shortens muscles in the back of your leg, called the hamstrings. Over time, muscles that stay in a shortened position for hours, days, or weeks, tend to stay in that shortened state. Imagine a cold piece of clay. When we knead clay, we warm it up. By adding the warmth and movement of our hands, the clay becomes flexible and malleable. Just like working with clay, massage therapists use their hands to warm your muscles. The large glute and hamstring muscles benefit from being warmed up. Massage increases circulation to short tight muscles allowing fresh blood and heat to lengthen and unwind the tissue.

If you'd prefer not to have your glute muscles massaged, ask your Licensed Massage Therapist to skip massaging your glutes.

If you like really deep work on your glutes, you may be interested to know, there exists a massage myth that says, *No pain. No gain.* That is not true with massage therapy. Skilled massage therapists understand the balance of deep massage and relaxation massage.

Some massage therapists will work on the glutes through the sheet using their hands in a soft fist to knead, kind of like making bread. Some will use their elbow to find the hot spots and release the tension. Some therapists work directly on the skin. As previously mentioned, if the sheet is moved to expose your skin, a secure drape is expected. Feel free to tuck or move the sheet if it feels loose.

You are always in control of your massage. Please communicate and offer feedback to your Licensed Massage Therapist at any time during the session about what feels good and what doesn't feel so good. Some massage therapists may seem psychic, but they are not. Your feedback is critical to the enjoyment of your session.

4. How will I feel after the session?

You can expect to feel peaceful and calm after your session. Clients report an overall feeling of well-being.

Now and then there are side effects from the massage. Yes, you'll be blissful and without a care in the world. However, the benefits of massage can change your body chemistry. You may feel tired, nauseous, or even muscle soreness. You are most likely not sick or injured. So what causes the weird symptoms?

The massage has improved your body's ability to eliminate waste. As a result, you may have a higher concentration of waste products in your bloodstream. This affects people differently. Having a snack, drinking some electrolytes, and/or drinking some water may help with feeling tired or nauseous.

Most massage therapists have no interest in making a client's muscles feel sore. If you experience muscle soreness after a massage, it feels more like muscle soreness after workout. Consider taking a hot shower, soaking in Epsom salt bath, sitting in a whirlpool or taking an easy walk for 10-15 minutes. Each of these recommended protocols will elevate your core temperature and warm your muscles, reducing the amount of soreness.

5. How often should I get a massage?

You can expect some feedback from your massage therapist offering an opinion on when to schedule your next session. If they don't make a recommendation, ask. Standard operating procedure is to receive a massage every two to four weeks. More often if you like!

There's an urban legend that Bob Hope got a massage every day of his life from 80 years old until he was almost 100. Truth is it wasn't every day, but it was often several times a week. He credits massage and other life choices for living a long healthy life.[47]

By adding massage therapy into your normal wellness routine, you will address current pain patterns and help control stress levels. Additionally, massage therapy will assist in preventing future injuries and managing stressful periods. If you are pain-free, wonderful. Massage will help to avoid problematic conditions and supplement a healthy lifestyle.

Once you experience a great massage, send your discoveries and insights to Jodi@JodiScholes.com. I love to read your stories about amazing massage/bodywork sessions!

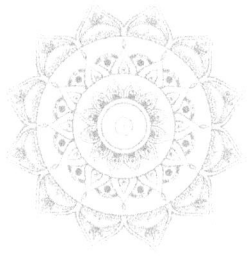

CHEAT SHEET

Did you know your body is telling your secrets?

Neck Pain

The message in neck pain is that you may be reluctant to see both sides of the story.

Shoulder Pain

Are you carrying the weight of the world on your shoulders? Let me be more specific. Do you have left shoulder pain? The left side of the body represents our feminine nature. If you have left-side shoulder pain, that leads me to ask, what feminine role are you in right now that you are beginning to resent? Do you have right-side shoulder pain? The right side of our body represents the masculine roles. What masculine role are you in right now, and are you starting to resent that role?

Low Back Pain

The low back is the area below the last rib and above the hip bones. Low back pain represents money. Too much, too little, this area is about the flow of money.

Want to dig a little deeper on this one? Left-side lower back pain leads to asking about feminine roles. Maybe you aren't contributing as much money to the household as you have in the past. Strong females tend to wrestle with seeing the value in staying at home. Not bringing home a paycheck. Spending money you didn't make. That internal dialogue can show up as pain on the left side of the lower back.

Right side low back pain? We are still talking about money but more masculine stereotypes. Are you the major breadwinner in your family? Whether you are or are not, how do you feel about that? Do you resent being stuck in a job because of the income? Are you okay with how much or how little you contribute to the household?

Right-side back pain (specifically in the general kidney area) leads me to ask if there has been a financial setback that you feel responsible for. Ah, maybe there is a female in your household earning more money than you. How do you feel about that? These scenarios lead to mental stress that can translate into right-side lower back pain.

Hip Pain

Hips represent our foundation. Our core beliefs. Our stability and what we know to be true. If someone betrays your trust, that can show up as hip pain. The right side of the body represents masculine energy. Who is the male or male energy in your life that is causing you to question your foundation? The left side of the body represents feminine energy. Who is the female or feminine energy in your life shaking you to the core?

Knee Pain

Knee pain? Knees symbolize bowing down. Bending of the will. Abandoning your own needs to serve others. Knee pain can make you physically unable to walk, run, carry groceries, or climb stairs. Knee pain puts you on the bench where you can't help.

Left side knee pain? What female are you bowing down to? What feminine energy are you bending your will to please? Right side knee pain? What male in your life are you always giving in to? What masculine energy is causing you to change your plans and act like it's okay? Are you always doing what he wants to do?

Ankle Pain

Ankles symbolize flexibility. Where are you being rigid in your decision-making? Where could you be more flexible? Bumps in the road will come. Those uneven, uncertain times when you really don't know how it will turn out. Ankle pain tells us to be more flexible. Release attachment to the outcome. Roll with it.

Foot Pain

Often foot pain tells us it is time to take the next step. I find it's often a major step, like moving the location of where we live or where we work. Foot pain can be present when there is the opportunity to move to a perceived higher level. Graduating from college and completing a program that qualifies you for a better position can spark an episode of plantar fasciitis or general foot pain.

Left foot pain? When is it time to take the next step regarding typically feminine roles? Do you have a role as a mother, grandmother, or daughter where it's time to take the next step? Time to walk away? Left foot pain reveals you are ready to release what doesn't serve you in a feminine role.

Right foot pain? What masculine role are you walking towards? What masculine role are you walking away from? In your masculine roles such as father, grandfather, or son, where do you see you are ready to take a baby step forward to create more peace, love, and joy for yourself?

Your body is telling your secrets. It's revealing how you really feel, even if you haven't said it out loud. Your internal dialogue shows up in the outer world. It's how your biography becomes your biology.

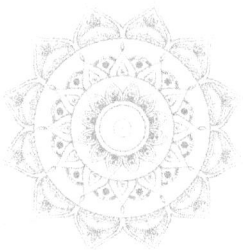

ENDNOTES

1   Dahlhamer J, Lucas J, Zelaya, C, et al. Prevalence of Chronic Pain and High-Impact Chronic Pain Among Adults — United States, 2016. MMWR Morb Mortal Wkly Rep 2018;67:1001–1006. DOI: http://dx.doi.org/10.15585/mmwr.mm6736a2. Accessed 3 January 2023.

2   Sullivan AR, Fenelon A. Patterns of widowhood mortality. J Gerontol B Psychol Sci Soc Sci. 2014 Jan;69(1):53-62. doi: 10.1093/geronb/gbt079. Epub 2013 Sep 27. PMID: 24077660; PMCID: PMC3968855. Web Accessed January 2023.

3   Borrell-Carrió F, Suchman AL, Epstein RM. The biopsychosocial model 25 years later: principles, practice, and scientific inquiry. Ann Fam Med. 2004 Nov-Dec;2(6):576-82. doi: 10.1370/afm.245. PMID: 15576544; PMCID: PMC1466742. Site visit August 2021

4   ibid

5   ibid

6   Brene Brown. "Daring Greatly: How the Courage to Be Vulnerable Transforms the Way We Live, Love, Parent and Lead." Avery: An imprint of Penguin Random House. 2012.

7   Ahuja V, Ranjan V, Passi D, Jaiswal R. Study of stress-induced temporomandibular disorders among dental students: An institutional study. Natl J Maxillofac Surg. 2018 Jul-Dec;9(2):147-154. doi:

10.4103/njms.NJMS_20_18.   PMID: 30546228;   PMCID: PMC6251286. Site visit 08/17/21

8   Stephen Kindler, et. al. "Depressive and Anxiety Symptoms as Risk Factors for Temporomandibular Joint Pain: A Prospective Cohort Study in the General Population." The Journal of Pain. November 9, 2012. Site visit August 17, 2021

9   Louise Hays "Heal Your Body A-Z: The Mental Causes for Physical Illness and the Metaphysical Way to Overcome Them." Hay House, Inc. 1998.

10   ibid.

11   Allissa Vitti. "WomanCode: Perfect Your Cycle, Amplify Your Fertility, Supercharge Your Sex Drive and Become a Power Woman." Harper One 2014.

12   Spencer S. Global Burden of Disease 2010 Study: A personal reflection. Glob Cardiol Sci Pract. 2013 Nov 1;2013(2):115-26. doi: 10.5339/gcsp.2013.15. PMID: 24689009; PMCID: PMC3963741. Site visit January 1, 2020.

13   Blozik E, Laptinskaya D, Herrmann-Lingen C, Schaefer H, Kochen MM, Himmel W, Scherer M. Depression and anxiety as major determinants of neck pain: a cross-sectional study in general practice. BMC Musculoskelet Disord. 2009 Jan 26;10:13. doi: 10.1186/1471-2474-10-13. PMID: 19171034; PMCID: PMC2636754. Site visit 01/01/20.

14   Cartoon graphic taken from https://condenaststore.com/featured/a-man-is-seen-sitting-in-an-oversized-snow-globe-felipe-galindo.html

15   N.A. "Headaches" Reduce stress to prevent the pain." N.D. the mayoclinic.org.

16   Eckhart Tolle. "The Power of Now: A Guide to Spiritual Enlightenment." August 19, 2004. New World Library.

17   Robert Plomin. "Behavior Genetics." February 11, 2019. Encyclopedia Britannica.

18   Edwin Chen. "Twins Reared Apart: A living lab." December 9, 1979. New York Times. Site visit November 12, 2022.

19   Stephanie Sciamento. "Why Do So Many Women Have Thyroid Disease?" Stephaniesciamento.com. ND. Site visit January 1, 2020.

20   Petar Mandincová. "Psychosocial Factors in Patients with Thyroid Disease". Thyroid and Parathyroid Diseases - New Insights into Some Old and Some New Issues, edited by Laura Ward, IntechOpen, 2012. 10.5772/36477.

21   https://www.stlukes-stl.com/health-content/medicine/33/000093. htm Site visit March 2023

22   Mary Ancillate. "9 Healing Crystals and Stones for the Throat Chakra (Vishuddha Chakra)" November 3, 2022. Angelgrotto.com.

23   Thorwald Dethlefsen and Dr. Rudiger Dahlke. "The Healing Power of Illness: Understanding What Your Symptoms Are Telling You" Vega. October 1, 2002. Site visit May 8, 2020.

24   Melanie Creedy. "Symbolism of Illness: Lungs & Breath." March 3, 2016. Elementsofhealth.com Site visit May 8, 2020.

25   Max Strom. "Breathe to Heal." TedxCapeMay. ND.

26   I enjoyed the blog by Judy Piazza of the Ojai Foundation/Topa Institute who wrote on her experience of a broken wrist. Site visit April 2023 https://www.youthpassageways.org/the-school-of-the-injured-wrist/

27   Siddhārtha Gautama. "The Life of the Buddha: Based on Original Sources" March 1, 2014. Real Reads.

28   Louise Hay. "Frequently Asked Questions." ND. Louisehay.com. Site visit August 22, 2021.

29   Mark Lord. "Forgiveness, the Direct Path to Love." Center for Spiritual Living. Seattle. February 22, 2015.

30   https://pubmed.ncbi.nlm.nih.gov/19539119/ Thank you for the research done by Elyse Shafarman for her article, "Jaw & Hip Connection." June 14, 2014. Bodyproject.com. Site visit April 10, 2023

31   Louise Hay. "Heal Your Body A-Z: The Mental Causes for Physical Illness and the Metaphysical Way to Overcome Them." Hay House, Inc. 1998.

32 Emily Francis. "The Body Heals Itself: How Deeper Awareness of Your Muscles and Their Emotional Connection Can Help You Heal." December 8, 2017. Llewellyn Publications. Site visit April 30, 2020.

33 Lo, Pei-Chia MD, MSa; LiLin, Fong-Cheng MDb; Tsai, Yao-Chien MD, MSc; Lin, Shun-Ku MD, MSc,d,∗. Traditional Chinese medicine therapy reduces the risk of total knee replacement in patients with knee osteoarthritis. Medicine 98(23):p e15964, June 2019.

34 Bark S. Ferket et. al. "Impact of total knee replacement practice: cost-effectiveness analysis of data from the Osteoarthritis Initiative" March 28, 2017. The National Library of Medicine: National Center for Biotechnology Information.

35 Katherine Woodward Thomas. "Conscious Uncoupling. Five Steps to Living Happily Even After." October 8, 2016. Harmony.

36 Lao Tzu. "Tao Te Ching (The Way) by Lao-Tzu: Special Collector's Edition with an Introduction by the Dalai Lama" January 1, 2011. NMD Books.

37 Jay Yarow. "AOL's CEO Makes His Executives Spend 10% Of Their Time Just Thinking Every Day." December 23, 2014. Business Insider.

38 Jeff Wiener. "The Importance of Scheduling Nothing." April 3, 2013. Linkedin.com.

39 N.A. "Why am I Breaking out in Hives when I'm Stressed? It's Probably not a Coincidence (or punishment)." March 7, 2019. Health Essentials. Clevelandclinic.org. Site visit January 25, 2021.

40 https://laurabruno.wordpress.com/2013/01/28/healthy-skin-a-medical-intuitive-perspective/ Site visit April 15, 2023

41 N.A. "Condition: Fibromyalgia." N.D. American Chronic Pain Association. tehacpa.org. Site visit Feb 5 2021.

42 https://pubmed.ncbi.nlm.nih.gov/11286669/ site visit April 16, 2023

43 N.A. "What Causes Fibromyalgia? Signs Point to Changes in the Brain." October 24, 2019. Health Essentials, Clevelandclinic.org. Site visit Dec 21, 2020.

44 N.A. "Drugs and Supplements Duloxetine (Oral Route)." N.D. Mayoclinic.org. Site visit March 2022

45 Edwene Gaines. "The Four Spiritual Laws of Prosperity: A Simple Guide to Unlimited Abundance." October 11, 2006. Gildan Media, LLC.

46 Marianne Williamson. *A Return to Love: Reflections on the Principles of "A Course in Miracles"* Full quote: "Our deepest fear is not that we are inadequate. Our deepest fear is that we are powerful beyond measure. It is our light, not our darkness that most frightens us. We ask ourselves, 'Who am I to be brilliant, gorgeous, talented, fabulous?' Actually, who are you not to be? You are a child of God. Your playing small does not serve the world. There is nothing enlightened about shrinking so that other people won't feel insecure around you. We are all meant to shine, as children do. We were born to make manifest the glory of God that is within us. It's not just in some of us; it's in everyone. And as we let our own light shine, we unconsciously give other people permission to do the same. As we are liberated from our own fear, our presence automatically liberates others."

47 Source: *The Free Library*. S.v. "Bob Hope and the fountain of youth." Retrieved Oct 06 2023 from https://www.thefreelibrary.com/ Bob+Hope+and+the+fountain+of+youth.-a03245216

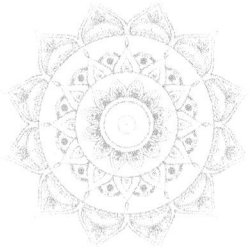

ABOUT THE AUTHOR

Jodi Scholes is a transformative healer and gentle teacher dedicated to guiding her clients and readers on a journey of self-understanding.

With over 25 years as a massage therapist and over 20,000 individual sessions, Jodi explains the body-mind connection. She empowers readers with knowledge of how to take the road less traveled, embracing vibrant well-being and living on purpose and pain-free.

Her time doing massage for professional athletes in soccer/ futbol, track & field, and triathlon fueled her curiosity about the root causes of pain and linking the connections between specific pain patterns and specific stressors.

Jodi's passion for sharing this message of wellness extends beyond her practice as she took the message to the TEDx stage sharing the experience with a global audience in 2021 based out of London.

She is an entertaining speaker, enthusiastic tennis player and aspiring foodie. She embraces an active life in the United States.

You can find her soaking up the great outdoors somewhere between Florida, Washington D.C. and New Hampshire.

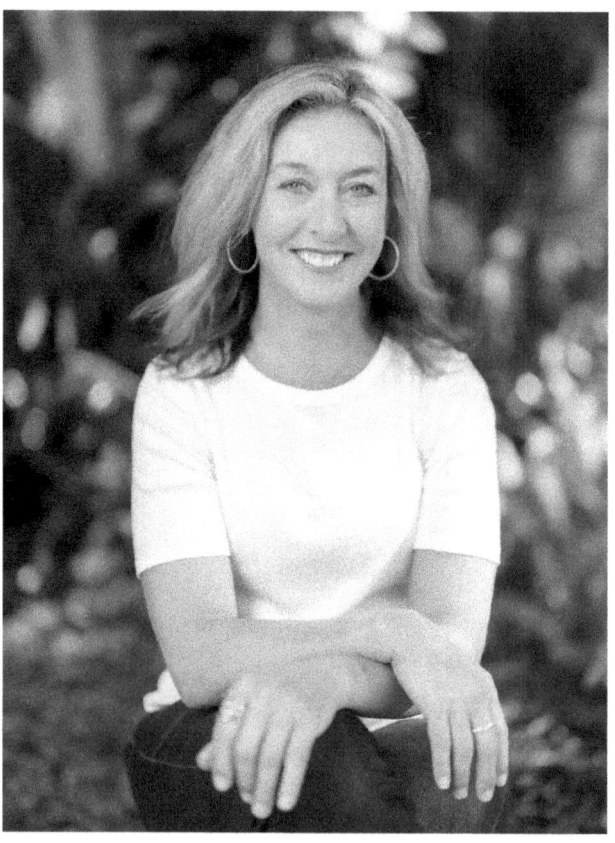

To learn more, join Jodi on a retreat that facilitates your own transformative journey or find out where she's speaking next, visit her website: JodiScholes.com.